Therapist as
Supervisor and Coach

Therapist as Supervisor and Coach

Gary A. Morse, M.A., M.S.

Consultant and Professional Coach and Trainer,
Morse & Associates, Colorado Springs, Colorado

with Forewords by

Larry P. Fronheiser, P.T.

Allegheny & Chesapeake Physical Therapists, Inc.,
Ebensburg, Pennsylvania

and

Julie O. Gardner, Ph.D., SLP
Diane S. Manzella, Ed.D., SLP

Gardner Manzella, Inc., Sherman Oaks, California

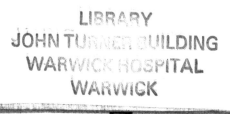
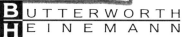

BUTTERWORTH
HEINEMANN

Boston Oxford Johannesburg Melbourne New Delhi Singapore

Every effort has been made to ensure that the drug dosage schedules within this text are accurate and conform to standards accepted at time of publication. However, as treatment recommendations vary in the light of continuing research and clinical experience, the reader is advised to verify drug dosage schedules herein with information found on product information sheets. This is especially true in cases of new or infrequently used drugs.

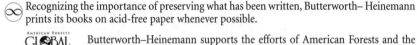
Library of Congress Cataloging-in-Publication Data

Morse, Gary A.
    Therapist as supervisor and coach / Gary A. Morse.
        p.   cm.
    Includes bibliographical references and index.
    ISBN 0-7506-7095-9 (alk. paper)
    1. Medical rehabilitation.   2. Physical therapist and patient.
    3. Therapist and patient.   I. Title.
    [DNLM: 1. Rehabilitation--methods.   2. Physical Therapy--methods.
    3. Occupational Therapy--methods.   4. Professional-Patient Relations.
    WB 320 M885t 1998]
    RM930.M68 1998
    610.69'6--dc21
    DNLM/DLC
    for Library of Congress   98-23837
                                                                        CIP

British Library Cataloguing-in-Publication Data
A catalogue record for this book is available from the British Library.

The publisher offers special discounts on bulk orders of this book.

For information, please contact: For information on all B-H medical
Manager of Special Sales   publications available, contact our
Butterworth–Heinemann   World Wide Web home page at:
225 Wildwood Avenue   http://www.bh.com
Woburn, MA 01801-2041
Tel: 781-904-2500
Fax: 781-904-2620

10 9 8 7 6 5 4 3 2 1

Printed in the United States of America

This book is affectionately dedicated to my mother Roberta, whose lifelong dream to touch others with her words was never fully realized.

Contents

Foreword I   xiii
Larry P. Fronheiser

Foreword II   xv
Julie O. Gardner and Diane S. Manzella

Preface   xvii

Acknowledgments   xxi

**I. New Skills for the New Environment: 1
    A Foundation**

  1 **A New Fork in the Road**   3
     The Golden Age
     A Very Revealing Survey
     Therapists Have Always Been Managers

  2 **Who Are You and What Do You   13
     Stand For?**
     Reflections
     Taking Inventory
     Personal Values, Professional Values, and Management
     A Personal Set of Management Principles
     Beaming with Balance

  3 **Relationship Management**   33
     The Empowerment Revolution
     Empowerment and Problem Solving
     The Control-Empowerment Dilemma
     A New Customer
     Humility and the Secondary Customer
     Organizational Structure: The Relationship
         of Company Relationships
     Safe and Proper Distance: Friendship and Work

The Organization as a Family: Asset or Liability?
Family of Origin and Health Care
Parent Trapping
The Molting Process

II. Performance!   **63**

4   **Expectation Alignment: An Ongoing Process**   **65**
What is Expectation Alignment?
Boundary Management
When Does Expectation Alignment Occur?

5   **Hiring: Finding the Fit**   **75**
Treatment as an Analogy
Pre-Interview Tips
Interviewing Tips
My Favorite Five: Tangential Questions That Evoke
    Interesting Answers
Group Interviews: Time Well Invested
Orientation Done Well
Off to a Great Start!

6   **Supervision and Coaching: Keeping the Fit**   **93**
Vision: Not Always So Super
Think Before You Help
Supervision Versus Coaching
Delegating with Grace
The Unforgivable Five: Terrible Transgressions Among
    Therapist-Supervisors
The Fabulous Five: Tried Tricks of the Trade
Final Thoughts for the Supervisor-Coach

7   **Performance Appraisal: Where It All**   **115**
Comes Together
A Tool, Not a Weapon
If It Is a Surprise, It Is a Symptom
Another Realignment Opportunity

Valuable Review Resources
Hard Copy
Amalgamation
Delivery
About Paper Trails . . .

8 **Vocational Divorce: When It Doesn't Work Out**   129
Corrective Action
Types of Separation
Resignation as an Option
The Termination Session
Turnover Rates
Divorce Done Well

III. It's About Time!   **137**

9 **Proper Focus**   139
Evolving Toward Self-Management
Doing What's Right: Urgency and Importance
Urgency Addiction

10 **Applied Time Management:**   153
The Pyramid of Proficiency
The Three Faces of Ease
A Final Peek at the Pyramid

IV. Meetings: Congregational   **171**
Communication

11 **The Most Expensive Hour of the Day**   173
What Rehabilitation Staff Say About Meetings
The Boredom Factor
Avoiding Total Failure

12 **Group Dynamics and Meeting Facilitation**   177
The "Group Movement"
Personal Evolution, Meeting Revelation

The Power of Numbers
Process Versus Content
Types of Group Meetings
Types of Outcomes
Process Happens

13   Creating Effective Meetings   **189**
Choose Members Carefully
The Almighty Agenda
Housekeeping
Ground Rules
Setting the Tone of a Meeting
Supervisor Spielberg
The Written Word
Dealing with Dysfunction
Closure
Closure, Part Two

V. *Confronting Conflict:*   **211**
**   *Tools for Turmoil***

14   Rehabilitation: Teeming with Teams   **213**
Multiple Disciplines, Multiple Skills
A Different Type of Identity Crisis
Being True to Your Team (to a Point . . .)

15   Nursing and the Therapies: Key Relationships   **221**
Professional Heritage
An Alien View
In Pursuit of the Proper Perspective
Reaching Out for Rationality

16   Conflict Consciousness   **241**
The "Yes" Culture
Emotional Capability of the Supervisor
Causes and Sources

17 Intervention   253
    Response to Conflict: Fight, Flight, or Insight?
    Strategic Diffusion
    Strategic Feedback
    Other Conflict Concepts

18 Post-Master (In the AfterTASC)   269

    Suggested Reading   273

Appendices   **275**

    1 Me and Supervision   277

    2 Key Incident Journal   279

    3 Structure of a Good Performance Appraisal   281
       Instrument in the Rehabilitation Industry

    4 Time Will Tell: A Self-Survey   289

    5 TASC Terms: The Language of Management   291
       and Supervision

Index   **303**

Foreword I

1998 marks my thirtieth year as a physical therapist. During those years I have practiced in a variety of settings: acute care hospitals, home care, extended care facilities, pediatric settings, and private practice. My education in the 1960s was clinically based, and, even today, the majority of education for physical therapists is rooted in the scientific basis of treatment techniques and successful clinical outcomes. In each clinical setting in which I rendered services, however, a significant part of my day was spent in activities for which I was relatively unprepared—management and supervision. I wish, at the start of my career, I had the book you are about to read, *Therapist as Supervisor and Coach*.

I first met Gary during my early years on the Board of Directors and worked with him recently in my current role as president of the National Association of Rehabilitation Agencies (NARA). He was a frequent presenter at NARA conferences, and his lectures, along with subsequent articles he wrote, left a significant impression on me as a therapist. His ability to understand the therapy professions so well, although not a therapist himself, is unique in terms of both his insight and foresight. After reading this book and enjoying the numerous anecdotal and researched examples of the author's management experience, you will feel as though you have spent several hours conversing with Gary. He knows and understands the needs of therapists who have been thrust into the supervisory and management arena. After reading this book, you should be able to enter your work environment and immediately apply the principles and knowledge Gary has shared.

The health care industry generally, and rehabilitation services specifically, are undergoing a major metamorphosis in the late 1990s. The challenges facing all of us as clinicians are significant; the challenges facing all of us as managers, supervisors, and coaches are critical to our success. Whether you are in your third or thirtieth year as a managing practitioner, you will enjoy and benefit from the experiences and ideas presented in this text.

Larry P. Fronheiser

Foreword II

The field of health care is in the midst of a period of volatile change fueled by back-to-back mandatory financial restructuring of Medicare by the Health Care Financing Administration. These changes affect the financial milieu of every company and person in health care today. The growth of health care maintenance organizations and the rapid consolidation and mergers of health care companies in an effort to increase productivity and efficiency have created opportunities for some and displacement and financial downsizing for others. As a result of the changing medical landscape, there has been a shift in decision making from management to the front line. This shift in authority is necessary in competitive markets such as health care, where delivery of service to the patient must be user friendly, competent, and timely. Management has taken on the new role of "servant leader" in acting as a resource to their staff. Management provides the vision and develops policy, but steps aside to let the people on the front line execute company policy.

A manager or supervisor in health care today has challenges that previous managers never faced. Modes of staffing can change rapidly with accompanying changes in salary structure. Therapists are forced to relocate to more distant geographic locations. Professional women, as well as men, are initiating relocations. More employees are seeking legal avenues to settle disputes. Restructuring creates stresses that can culminate in legal claims of perceived mismanagement. Managerial skills can be tested by conflict in dealing with professional sharing of capitated therapy minutes or funds. Managers must read newspapers daily to stay on the cutting edge of health care, to anticipate and proactively meet goals. In a world where most people, young and old, seek predictability and stability, corporate entities must constantly restructure to remain viable. Managers must be able to shift rapidly and prepare employees to do the same. Employees are reacting to this volatility by placing more emphasis on their personal fulfillment and family life, over which they have more control, and less emphasis on loyalty to their employers.

Few therapist-managers have MBAs. Most have learned by trial and error or by emulating someone thought to be a good manager. New therapist-managers are usually chosen because of their skillful self-management and confidence in professional skills and communication. In most professional therapy programs, the curriculum does not include instruction or required reading in therapy management. Such training is long overdue. Therapist-managers have to develop the skills to cope with the array of complex problems facing the deliverers of therapy services in today's environment of decreased financial support.

In *Therapist as Supervisor and Coach*, Gary Morse has created an outstanding guide and reference that every managing therapist should have. It offers wonderful pearls of wisdom to keep a manager out of trouble legally and professionally. The book covers the wide scope of topics necessary to today's therapy delivery systems. As a bonus, the book was written with practical examples from real-life situations, for ease of assimilation and application. The book has the potential not only to improve therapist-manager skills, but also to make therapists the best therapist-managers they can become.

Julie O. Gardner
Diane S. Manzella

Preface

A Treatment of Another Sort

This is not just another book on management. This one is for you, the therapist: occupational, physical, or speech and language. It is also for you, the assistant, who is often asked to supervise an aide or a tech (if your state so allows). What distinguishes this book from the others is focus. The lens here is pointed at line staff charged with supervisory duties in a rehabilitation setting. The assumption is that you have not had training and formal experience—at least not in the rehabilitation world—and that you want it. A further difference is context. The complex work arrangements, team dynamics, and interdependent peer relationships that are esoteric to our corner of the health care industry demand a special approach; thus, the strategies discussed here are taken from real-life, clinically based scenarios, lived out by you and your peers daily. No lofty tome of management theory, this volume operates in the time-tried trenches of rehabilitation.

One would hope that no legitimate institution (hospital, nursing home, clinic, or school) would send an untrained, unlicensed therapist out to evaluate and treat a patient or client. Yet rehabilitation organizations nationwide expect untrained therapists and assistants to supervise and coach subordinates without special preparation. In most cases, it is only when one is already employed in a titled management position that formal supervisory training begins, if ever. I have spoken with therapists about this dilemma for years, and the opinion appears to be universal across the country: The industry needs a book, a guide on how to supervise and coach. You are holding that book.

Reading this book will not lead to formal certification, but it will give you a solid foundation. If you are still in school, it will prepare you for what you might expect on the floors of American rehabilitation institutions. If you are a veteran therapist, it will remind you of those times you struggled with a performance appraisal or juggled a half-dozen crises at once, lacking both the time and the tools to respond effectively. If you are a manager, it will challenge you to arm your therapists and assistants with the proper skills and tools to supervise.

The industry is undergoing the most tumultuous period in its history. Diminishing revenues will further deplete the ranks of middle management, placing increased pressure on therapists to be innovative and productive. The ability to supervise, heretofore an afterthought for most therapists, will be elevated to new levels in the new environment, and you must embrace this challenge *now.*

I am an organizational psychologist and physiologist by training, and a health care administrator, writer, coach, and organizational consultant by practice. The first 20 years of my career were spent managing in the mental health field, with particular emphasis on chemical dependency; the past 8 years have been focused on physical rehabilitation in acute hospital, outpatient, long-term care, and home-care environments. For the past 12 years, I have shared many of the thoughts and ideas in this book through workshops, newsletter columns, and other media. I find that therapists are increasingly eager to learn about management and supervision.

You will notice a consistent management philosophy throughout this book. Much of it has formal academic underpinnings, but most of it comes from the school of hard knocks. You won't find many $50 management terms here, because they don't serve the purpose. You want everyday answers to everyday problems.

In studies and in practice, I have attempted to embrace motivational theory, group dynamics, organization-family models, and athletic coaching analogies as principal guideposts, with a fundamental respect for human-to-human love as a thematic foundation. Management, supervision, and coaching are about relationships, be they between two people or 20. The job here is to clarify those relationships, bring them into alignment, and accomplish what you and the organization want: successful outcomes and happy employees.

So there you have it. This is a treatment of a different sort: supervision and coaching in rehabilitation. I hope you find this book to be helpful and that your practice is successful.

G.A.M.

Acknowledgments

I believe that behind every good project is a good family, and mine is wonderful, not to mention *patient*. Thanks to Kellyn, Devin, and Barbara (my wife and personal editor) for tolerating my rantings at Windows 95 and its strange idiosyncrasies. Also, many thanks to Karen Selley, OTR, whose brilliance as a leader and thinker is matched only by her thoughtfulness as a friend. Warm regards to my two Marys (Dwan and Twinem), the soul sisters who encouraged me to be myself and to pursue my dreams as a writer. Finally, to Dot Smith I owe both thanks and undying respect, for her inspiration and unparalleled professionalism.

For technical content, I wish to acknowledge the American Speech and Hearing Association, the University of Iowa (Wendell Johnson Speech Pathology and Audiology Department), Bethel College of Nursing at the University of Colorado at Colorado Springs, the National Association of Rehabilitation Agencies, and the Webb Library at Penrose Hospital in Colorado Springs.

Last but not least, I thank all of the therapists, assistants, technicians, teachers, and nurses with whom I have worked in this incredible field of medicine. We who know what you do each day share your passion for improving the human condition. You are to be admired for your dedication and skill. I hope that this book is a contribution to your comfort and effectiveness as a supervisor and coach.

G.A.M.

I   New Skills for the New Environment: A Foundation

As we enter a new era in the field of rehabilitation, new skills will be required. Licensed therapists have been asked to supervise one, two, or perhaps three aides or assistants in the past; the new environment could grow that number to five, six, or even seven. External forces will increase the number of care extenders, exert additional pressure on productivity, and demand better outcomes with less reimbursement. Middle management will shrink in numbers, bringing increased responsibility for managerial effectiveness to the staff therapist level. In other words, you will have not just one job but two: You are the therapist-supervisor.

Just as you sought basic training in your chosen discipline, you must now seek it in supervision and coaching. There are many interesting parallels between therapy and management, and if you look for them, you can fully exploit the talent and experience you already have as a trained therapist. Rehabilitation is, after all, a service business, and much of management is the business of serving the employees who work under your supervision.

There are several differences between a solid foundation in an area of emphasis and *splinter skills*. Splinter skills are gained when learning occurs in an episodic fashion: event by event, person by person, without any grounding in theory or principle. Splinter skills may be easier to apply at the time, but they don't transcend settings or situations well, and they usually result in fragile, short-term solutions. Foundational skills, on the other hand, emanate from a grounded philosophy that has stood the test of time. They tend to produce consistency and reliability with more predictable results.

This first section helps you to take a look at yourself, your industry, and your peers in the context of supervision. Data show that you are not drawn to managerial practice by nature, yet you know what you want in an effective manager. It is hoped that the philosophic basis of good management practice—included in the latter half of the section—will launch you on the road toward *becoming* that effective manager.

1
A New Fork in the Road

A Look at What You'll Learn:

- Why things are changing after the golden age of rehabilitation
- How the arrival of the "work-site shuffle" has affected our jobs
- Why there are new challenges and a call for new skills among therapists
- The priorities of therapists, assistants, and managers, according to a survey of rehabilitation staff
- Therapy and supervision: similar skills with a different focus

The Golden Age

Wasn't it marvelous! After decades of struggling to become recognized, reimbursed, and reinforced, we finally nailed it in the mid-1980s. The Omnibus Budget Reconciliation Act (OBRA) of 1984 passed, insurance companies woke up, we figured out how to play the Medicare game, and therapy went wild. Rehabilitation agencies grew like wildflowers, schools sprouted new professional programs, and salaries skyrocketed. New training institutes arose everywhere, durable medical equipment (DME) sales went bananas, and the suppliers filled the trade magazines with ads from cover to cover. First it was physical therapy, then occupational, and finally speech, and the industry was on a roll. There was such a shortage of therapists that the media actually described it as a health care crisis. Rehabilitation's golden age lasted from 1985 to 1995.

Then some not-so-fun things started to happen. Managed care lurched further forward and started the squeeze, often restricting treatments to five or six sessions in their now-familiar standardized mandates. Operation Restore Trust kicked in, and the FBI made a few surprise visits to therapists to investigate fraud and abuse. A therapist in Colorado actually went to prison. Doctors started getting a little tight, and fearing overutilization, they began withholding orders. Salary equivalency loomed above occupational therapy and speech, and focused reviews of records became almost the norm. Then came the big blow to those treating Medicare patients: the Budget Reconciliation Act of 1997, with new limits on outpatient therapies, prospective payments in home care and long-term care, and a government-driven downsizing of the industry.

Clearly, the *industry* is adjusting as we look toward the new century. What about you, the practitioner? What has happened to you in the midst of all this change? In the early 1990s, you and your peers were comfortably nestled in hospitals (for the most part), aiming your 8 hours at strokes and hips in the rehabilitation units, with an occasional stint for the acute bedside team on another floor. If you weren't doing inpatient care, you were busy treating workers' compensation injuries and weekend warriors in the outpatient clinic at a nice pace of 8–10 patients a day. Salaries continued to rise, and benefits were among the best in the country. There seemed to be no end to the increase in stature and compensation.

Then came the mass migration to long-term care. Subacute units gutted the hospital rehabilitation beds, outpatient clinics opened in skilled nursing facilities (SNFs), and half the nursing home chains in the country bought their own rehabilitation companies to take advantage of the wide-open Medicare regulations for geriatric rehabilitation. The meteoric rise of salaries was tempered a bit, and benefits began to level as all eyes turned toward Washington. We held our collective breath as the list of threats grew: whistle-blowing, salary equivalency, prospective payment, limits on Medicare B, and managed Medicare.

In 1996, the "work-site shuffle" began. Hospitals, rehabilitation companies, and nursing homes began to diversify to keep therapists productive. They looked everywhere for new business: home care, group homes, assisted-living centers, retirement communities, even shopping malls. Instead of treating in a single setting, many therapists began running around town, doing a home-care visit here, an

SNF treatment there, with perhaps a quick stop at the outpatient clinic before returning to the home office to complete four types of documentation forms—two of which they had never seen before. With little or no training in time management, most therapists ended their days far behind, feeling disorganized and discouraged, pining for the old days of 70% productivity.

Not a pretty picture. Not pretty, but not unusual either. Whether we like it or not, the country could not bear the cost of so much high-cost therapy, so it adjusted. It adjusted through managing workers' compensation, commercial health insurance, personal injury protection (PIP) plans, Medicaid, and Medicare with aggressive measures. Actually, we were just a few years behind the physicians (with a golden age of their own, roughly 1975–1985), whose industry had become overspecialized and costly and whose wings were cut by legislation and managed care in the late 1980s and early 1990s. The doctors hated it. They yelled and screamed and threatened anarchy, but guess what: They changed. They grouped their practices, punted many tasks to nurses, joined health maintenance organizations (HMOs), and became aggressive managers of their practices. Yes, there were casualties. A psychiatrist friend of mine dropped completely out of the hospital and insurance melee and now takes only private pay patients—nice if you can do it, but hardly the answer for most physicians or therapists. The rest of us mortals must learn new skills to allow us to fully use our old knowledge.

Our industry must react. There *will* be rehabilitation. We *will* survive. Our therapy is simply too effective to just disappear from the health care scene like dust in the wind. New treatment models will arise, new partnerships will evolve, and the system will adjust. Meanwhile, you as an individual must make your own personal adjustment. You need to become more organized. You must run meetings efficiently. You need to know how to handle conflict. You need to develop even stronger relationships with nonrehabilitation peers. You need to know how to supervise, to amplify your impact. And you need to know more about yourself as a person performing a dual role.

A Very Revealing Survey

In 1996, Cheyenne Mountain Therapies, Inc. (CMT) of Colorado Springs, Colorado, conducted a survey of physical, occupational, and speech therapists in an effort to better understand attitudes toward several issues related to management. Although the instrument was not scientifically validated, it was pretested, and the results were surprisingly consistent.

Because the work done by CMT was primarily in the geriatric arena, the distribution of the survey instrument was somewhat oriented to professionals working in long-term care; however, with the possible exception of the "less than 4 years' experience" group, most therapists had worked in multiple settings, including hospitals, outpatient clinics, and home care. Moreover, the student population was not biased in this fashion, none having actually worked as a therapist in a single rehabilitation environment at the time of the survey.

A total of 332 surveys were returned from 11 states, with questions asked of the following groups:

- Students (affiliate level)

- Staff therapists (<4 years' experience; 4–6 years' experience; and >6 years' experience)

- Assistants* and aides

- Rehabilitation managers

Each survey was tailored to the target group, and the number of questions (mostly rank-order choices) ranged from four to eight. In essence, the survey sought information on the following issues:

- Reasons for becoming a therapist

- Concerns (or fears) on entering the field of therapy

- Ranking of challenges faced by therapists

---

*Physical therapist assistants (PTAs) and certified occupational therapy assistants (COTAs) are hereinafter referred to as "assistants."

- Skills necessary for success as a therapist
- Degree of training and experience in managing/supervising
- Level of importance placed on personally having management/supervision skills
- Chosen topics if therapist was designing a management/supervision course for therapists
- Most important roles played by a therapist
- Biggest surprises in working as a therapist

Several things were immediately apparent upon the tabulation of results. First, therapists and therapy students are not fundamentally oriented toward management and supervision when those choices are ranked against other more clinically based items. In fact, management/supervision was consistently the *last* choice by a fairly wide margin. The orientation of professionals in this field begins with and remains with the *patient* in a hands-on relationship. There is no doubt about what most of you came to do: therapy. Furthermore, supervising and giving direction to others is *not* seen as a primary concern, challenge, or role by students or practicing therapists. Not surprisingly, respondents again ranked these manager-like tasks at the bottom of their choice lists.

You may wonder what your peers *are* concerned about. The answers: clinical judgment, managed care, and documentation. Organizing work time was a distant fourth, and, as inferred earlier, "supervising assistants/aides" was last. In the traditional environment, these priorities make sense. If you make poor clinical choices, you lose your license. Fail to please managed care, you lose future referrals. Deal with too much documentation, you lose your mind. However, if you fail to supervise your assistants and aides adequately, you could lose all of those things a lot faster.

When veteran therapists and therapy managers were asked to prioritize things that proved to be surprises in their work experience, the responses were similar to those chosen as major concerns.

"Productivity requirements" was an additional item that ranked high as a surprise, alluding to the fact that the infamous *P*-word plagues us all. "Having to supervise others" ranked last among the surprises, indicating that most therapists knew that they would be supervising someone when they entered the field. Even so, it appears that this function—supervising—gets lost in the shuffle in the rush to prove one's self clinically and rarely gets equal time in the minds of most therapists.

With regard to management/supervision training and experience, three queries were made:

1. How much training have you had in managing/supervising other people? (Choices: considerable, some, very little, none)

2. How much experience have you had in managing/supervising other people? (Choices: considerable, some, very little, none)

3. What level of importance would you place on management/ supervision skills in terms of being a successful staff therapist? (Choices: of no importance, minor, moderate, or great importance)

About 50% of the students and therapists reported "some" training, whereas "considerable" training totaled 6% and 11%, respectively. Interestingly enough, the managers reported only 6% under "considerable" and 47% under "some."

Rankings of the importance of management training were encouraging to me. Approximately 90% of students, therapists, and managers thought that such training was of moderate or great importance. I thought it significant that 72% of the assistant/aide respondents found management training to be of "great" importance, a not-so-subtle message from those who had been supervised by ill-prepared therapists in the past.

Finally, the question was asked, "If you were designing a management/supervision course specifically for therapists, which of the following three topics would you choose for their value in the current work environment? Please *circle* your top choice:"

- Facilitating meetings
- Conflict resolution
- Time management
- Performance evaluation/appraisal
- Goal setting
- Leadership skills
- Other (_____)

With the exception of "facilitating meetings" (which scored the lowest), the six skills listed garnered a relatively even distribution of scores. "Conflict resolution" and "time management" were the top choices, with "leadership skills" a close third. The fact that "facilitating meetings" scored significantly lower is perhaps reflective of the degree of disdain most of us have for meetings in general. More on that later.

Taken as a whole, the results of this survey helped mold the design of my Therapist as Supervisor workshops and this book. I have taken the time to review the data because it helps to validate some of the challenges facing therapists. Without an inclination toward management training, licensed therapists are left with the dilemma that has plagued many other service industries in the past: learning by doing.

Therapists Have Always Been Managers

When you think about it, therapists have always had to juggle a number of balls at once: patients, families, documentation, special projects, supervisees, supply ordering, and continuing education, just to name a few. Your work life has become much more complicated, and keeping all the balls in the air is a daily challenge. If you work in a multidisciplinary setting, you are constantly managing relationships:

making sure the director of nursing (DON) is happy, keeping the team from alienating the nurses, trying to stay in tune with dietary needs and social work and activities, trying to stay close to maintenance so they will fix the wheelchairs, and so on. Even finding the time to go to the bathroom is a challenge!

In clinical work you constantly make judgments. You screen, assess, set goals, treat, grade the activity, discharge, take a breath, and start over again with another patient or client. In between the screens and discharges, you cheerlead, collaborate, challenge, cajole, and celebrate when gains are made. Many relationships—some close, some distant— are wrought and wrangled in the process without much notice, because this is the game of rehabilitation, and you play it every day.

There are many parallels to this clinical script in supervision and coaching. You are constantly judging subordinate staff. The touchy-feely types of the world would like to say that we should not judge others, but in fact, we do. Constantly. It goes with the territory. Admittedly, the emphasis of your judgment is more toward personality, attitude, and relationships, but in the end it is all about performance. Isn't that what we look for and judge in our patients— performance? Don't we have to evaluate cognitive ability, compliance, follow-through, and outcomes in the clinical sense every day? Don't we then document all of this carefully, comparing outcomes with goals, justifying what we did?

Your clinical skills can easily transfer to supervisory skills. You are not some dummy off the street. You are used to focusing, thinking quickly, developing relationships, evaluating situations and people, recording your thoughts on paper (or on computer), and performing as a professional. In the ensuing sections, we will add a few new wrinkles to that existing set of skills.

MORSELS

In the CMT survey, when assistants and aides were asked to select the top three skills needed by their supervising therapists, they chose, in order, (1) ability to listen, (2) approachability, and (3) ability to make decisions. Other responses indicated that therapists must seek better ways to provide access to their supervisees, who want to be heard and understood. These are the primary challenges for anyone in a management-related role; without the skills to meet such basic challenges, a supervisor cannot move forward to more sophisticated endeavors.

2

Who Are You and What Do You Stand For?

A Look at What You'll Learn:

- How you really feel about yourself in the leadership role
- Where your personal and professional values intersect
- A useful list of proven management principles
- The pursuit of balance in your work life
- Useful tips for handling stage fright

Reflections

In training supervisors, I have found it instructive to ask them to go back over their lives in search of events that relate to the task at hand. Sit back for a moment, close your eyes if you wish, and take a moment to think about you . . .

What is your first memory associated with being in a leadership role? How old were you? Was it at school, in church, or did it have something to do with the family? Was it student council, perhaps, or some kind of committee? An athletic team? The point guard, running the floor? Maybe it was later, in college, or in your first job. When was that first time?

How did it feel to be cast in the role of the leader? Were you ready for it? Did it scare you? Were you overcome with dread for the responsibility of being the person in charge? Did you have to speak in front of an audience? Were you confident? Did you like the feeling of being in an adultlike role as a kid? Did the experience lead you to seek other leadership roles or cause you to shy away from similar pursuits?

Such reflection is useful for several reasons. First, people often forget early traumas related to leadership that linger, acting as barriers to their progress. This is particularly true of public speaking, which many people automatically associate with management. Stage fright (panic anxiety, basically) is surprisingly widespread in the population, and many people hold themselves back from management positions for fear of having to speak in public. Even with all of the public speaking I do currently, I had a horrendous time with this about 20 years ago. Several embarrassing on-stage experiences occurred during the same year, leaving me fearful of speaking in front of more than two people at a time. I worked my way through the crisis, learned a few tricks of the trade (among presenters), and moved on. If presenting makes you feel a little shaky, see the Morsels at the end of this chapter for a few tips on how to combat stage fright.

Another reason for focused reflection is to understand your own comfort zone. I recently supervised two program coordinators, each of whom was responsible for about six other staff. Both had excellent instincts, great people skills, and fine intelligence. They were in entry-level management positions, and both would make fine managers, if not future administrators. The problem was one of them didn't *like* management. She loved to put her hands on patients, didn't want the extra burdens of management, and knew it. I thought that was great. The other woman *did* like management, *did* like supervision, and *did* stay on that career path. I loved and respected both of them for knowing what they did well and why.

If you are a therapist or an assistant, you might not have much choice about the matter. Supervision might well be part of the job, especially as we move into the twenty-first century. However, there *are* choices. In some corners of the business, you can be a single practitioner and avoid supervising anyone. In schools, you are less likely to have a formal supervisory role, although you will undoubtedly be working with volunteer aides and parents. For the rest (which is the majority), best belly up to the bar. The more you know about management and supervision, the more valuable you will be. The current prediction is that there will be a surplus of therapists by 2004, and you will want to possess every ounce of skill you can muster to be able to compete for jobs.

In any event, it is valuable to know yourself and your tendencies. In several places in this book, I will ask you to look inward before moving outward. Part of my goal is to help you develop a relationship with yourself—particularly your professional self. If you are fearful, this book will help you to work through the fear. So often many of us motor along in life, doing the same things, living out our patterned scripts, rarely stopping to say, "Why am I doing this?" Instead, we knee jerk with, "Oh well, that's the way I've always done it!" If you have had counseling, so much the better, because you'll know more about who you really are. If you are married—or better yet, have kids—that's an even bigger step forward; no one tells you more about who you really are than the spouse and children in your own home. It is rare that you gather such feedback at work.

Taking Inventory

In Appendix 1, you will find a short personal inventory called "Me and Supervision." It is a sentence-completion approach, aimed at getting you to think about yourself and some of your attitudes toward supervision and management. Take it now; it will help prepare you for the next few chapters.

Personal Values, Professional Values, and Management

Have you ever tried to distinguish between your personal and professional values? It's hard, isn't it? Ideally, they should be the same, but at times you find yourself compromising your personal values to be able to maintain your professional role. A good example is fighting with a managed care organization (MCO) over treatment duration. When you know in your heart that a patient needs at least 12 visits to be able to walk safely and the MCO says you're limited to six, both your personal and professional values are violated. On the other hand, the professional wisdom you have gained tells you that if you don't compromise sufficiently, you (or your company) won't be around to do the work anyway. Even worse, if the MCO develops a bad attitude toward rehabilitation, lots of people might not get therapy. This reviolates your personal-professional goal, which is to help people in need.

Management also has its principles. These principles might be described as values or philosophies in the various books that line the store shelves, but at the bottom of it all, they are core standards applied to a specific discipline. In fact, they are not that different from the practice acts that guide your work. The therapists who preceded you helped formalize the application of technique, and these doctrines were then formalized by the professional associations into practice acts. There are similar authorizing agencies in higher management (e.g., the American Management Association), but few (that I know of) at the line-staff level for the purpose of day-to-day supervision.

A Personal Set of Management Principles

In 28 years of management, I have begun to figure out what works; not just the management strategies—that is, the operational techniques described in the later sections—but the basic belief system that drives what I do. Because I have been in the service industry all of these years, I know that these principles translate down the line to the product that is provided to the ultimate customer. A work system that lacks guiding management principles is like the proverbial ship without a rudder. I call my own list a personal mission statement for the manner in which I manage myself and the work of other people. The following is my list of eight management values.

Honoring the Golden Rule

How basic can you get? You don't have to be religious to comprehend the power of the Golden Rule—you just have to be respectful of yourself and others. Any halfway-adjusted human being wants to be treated equally and fairly, and simply turning the tables in your mind is a fairly easy process, *if you pause long enough to consider that option*. Too many of us are quick to the draw—assuming that someone else is either stupid, malicious, or lazy—without taking the time to think about motives. I see it happen constantly, and it astounds me. Just put yourself in the other guy's place. It's that simple.

A couple of years ago I got caught in one of those ugly triangles that are often wrought by poor teamwork and failure to honor the Golden Rule. A speech-language pathologist (SLP) under my supervision in a nursing home began abusing the time of an aide who had been assigned to her because of a physical disability that prevented the therapist from driving. When the therapist began requesting that personal shopping on work time be included in the support she received, the aide balked and reported the incident to two other staff members; the information was promptly passed along to me. Meanwhile, the SLP abruptly stopped using her assigned aide, began using another one for rides between facilities, and made no mention of any changes to me. Needless to say, when I brought these two ladies together, venom was spewing across the table in both directions, and I ended up writing up the therapist after a confrontational counseling session.

You can extract at least three or four violations of the Golden Rule from this story. First, the SLP would not appreciate a demand to shop on *her* work time, yet she did that very thing to another staff member. Second, were the situation reversed, the aide would probably not enjoy knowing that such a story had spread around the team (an act she had herself accomplished quite thoroughly) by having it discussed with peers; the supervisor and *only* the supervisor should have been notified. Finally, in retaliation for the resistance from the first aide, the SLP dropped her for another aide, notifying neither her supervisor *nor* the first aide. This caused significant hassles for four people: both aides, the second aide's supervising therapist, and me. The details aren't necessarily the stuff of everyday problems, but the theme is: Do unto others as you would have them do unto you.

Keeping One's Integrity Intact

Webster defines *integrity* as "the quality or state of being of sound moral principle." I call it being true to one's values. Associated concepts include honesty, virtue, and righteousness. I would toss *fairness* onto the pile, although the evaluation of fairness is really in the eyes of the beholder.

You can't just *tell* people that you are honest and righteous, you must *show* them. You must demonstrate your consistent dedication to doing what is right, over and over again, to gain their trust and respect. In dozens of exit interviews over the years, I have heard departing employees comment about those special supervisors who had managed to maintain their integrity on the job. "She was always fair to me," they would say, or, "I could always depend on him to be honest with me." People never forget a fair shake, and in this business, "what goes around comes around" is especially true because we tend to run across former colleagues in new settings all the time. Jobs may come and go, but personal integrity will prevail. I have seen (more than once) rehabilitation staff follow supervisors from one company to another, just for the sake of that supervisor's personal integrity.

Keeping one's integrity intact is a constant challenge in management—particularly in middle management. As a therapist-supervisor you might not carry an official middle management title, but in essence you *are* a middle manager, because you're stuck between forces: line-level assistants and aides on one side and your own manager on the other. You will find your values tested regularly by conflicts that place you in the middle: Should you terminate that COTA that you feel has been misunderstood by upper management? Is it proper to keep that veteran rehabilitation aide at the same salary, while bringing on a kid for a dollar more an hour just because the team is desperate for help? Should you defend your program manager for the sake of the team, even though you disagree with the way she does her job? The list never ends.

I cannot honestly say that I have maintained my integrity in all supervisory situations. There were times when I yielded, compromised, and bent with the pressure to comply. However, honesty has always been very close to my heart, and if nothing else I want to go home at night feeling that I have been as fair as possible during the day.

Valuing Teams and Teamwork

The whole really *is* greater than its parts. There are few professions that demand more team participation than rehabilitation. It's almost as if *therapy* and *teamwork* are synonymous. A team can be as small as a therapist and an aide, or as large as a multidisciplinary group around the Medicare meeting table, where nurses, therapists, assistants, aides, social workers, recreational therapists, dietary aides, and physicians review the progress of a Medicare A caseload. Unless you are in a unique position in the industry (and I can't think of many), it is imperative that you value teams and teamwork.

As a manager, I value teams for many reasons. First, I love the camaraderie that occurs when a team steeps itself in problem solving. It's fun, it's exciting, and it can be very productive. There is something special about walking out of a great team meeting where much was accomplished, feeling that everyone has contributed something useful. It is a high that only fellowship can produce.

I also like the quality of work that teams produce. Team-generated ideas are usually better ideas. Because the group spawned them, action plans tend to get carried out quicker and more effectively. Different perspectives produce better solutions to tough problems.

In many rehabilitation settings, you work in an extended team situation. For example, in a hospital setting you might have your therapy team localized in a large collegial charting room, but the real rehab is done all over the building: at bedside with nursing, in the dining room with dietary, over the phone with the lab, in a conference room with a physician. If you are unable to balance your "piece of the patient" with other professionals, you are doing a disservice. You absolutely *must* have good listening skills, good chart-reading skills (a lost art, I believe), the ability to integrate your opinions, and the humility to back off at the right time.

Valuing teams means honoring the process of team building. Teams, like good wines, take time to mature; they go through stages and can be painfully ineffective at times. Sometimes they feel less like teams than clinical battlegrounds. Too many times, I have seen young therapists waltz into teams that are in the formative stages and behave as if everything should be working like clockwork. It just doesn't happen that way. Part of being a good team player is recognizing the maturity level of the group as an evolving entity itself; within that you need to assess the skills of the group's members, as well as where you sit on the power curve within that particular team. You might have enormous influence on one team (e.g., the speech team) and very little effect on another (e.g., the extended rehabilitation team in an SNF). You will sit quietly with your peers and be lectured by the medical director at 8:30 AM, only to lead a session on e-stim for your three charges (a PTA and two aides) at 10:00. That's the way it goes: give and take, yin and yang.

Team building doesn't just come from the top, it comes from all sides. Every fight, every success, every loss, and every gain contributes to what the team will become. Good teamwork needs not only good leaders, but good followers. In fact, it is often the behavior of the collective followers that best defines the success of the leaders. You will see tons of books on leadership, but few on followership. When you put a microscope to a good team, you often find that there are leaders among the followers. They might not be the ones standing, presenting, or carrying the torch to upper management, but they are there, supporting, reinforcing, and regularly making the ostensible leader's impact more effective. In other words, good followership is just good leadership at another level. Or, maybe, good leadership in another way. *It takes a conscious effort to be a good follower, and we are all followers somewhere in our lives.*

My final comment on teamwork has to do with commitment. If you really want to be a successful therapist-supervisor, you must be steadfast in your commitment to teamwork. That means that you plan, you listen, you respond, you compromise when appropriate, you follow up, and you look at the big picture. Sometimes you will be the quarterback calling the plays, and sometimes you will be on the bench; it doesn't matter, you are still on the team.

Being an Integrated Person

This is one of my favorite topics. For years, as I worked my way up through the ranks of management, I felt like two people: the at-home Gary and the at-work Gary. A certain tightness arose between the shoulder blades on the way to work each day, but I just ignored it and went my way, gearing up to be Gary at work. It seemed that the higher I went in management, the greater the knot behind the neck became, and the more I felt less like myself at work.

Then I went to work for my first real mentor. He was a wonderful man, an MD-MBA whom I will call Dr. S. This man had enormous responsibilities and endless talent. But it wasn't his talent that taught me, it was his *demeanor*. Dr. S walked from home, to work, to play with a fluidity that I had never seen before in someone with such pressure to perform. He was rarely in a bad mood, always had nice things to say to everyone, and was an inspirational figure to hundreds of his coworkers. How did he manage this?

It took me about 2 years to figure that out. The Great Doctor (a general practitioner, by the way) had become an *integrated* person. He had congruency in his lifestyle. He had decided that he liked what he did, that his personality served him well, and that he was not about to live two lives. He was funny, creative, loving, brilliant, supportive, interested, and interesting, but most of all, he was fluid. He functioned in many circles as the same person. What you saw was what you got; no funny business, no posturing, no phoniness.

Not all of us, including me, are as internally unified as my mentor friend. However, we can all makes steps toward integration. I did.

In watching Dr. S, I began to let more of myself out at work. I used family stories as metaphors when coaching my staff. I let my sense of humor diffuse crises at work, because that had always worked for me in my other walks of life. I comforted my people at work when they were hurting, just as I would my own children at home. Gradually, week by week, the knot contracted, and eventually went away.

About now, you are probably saying, "I can't do that! *My* job just won't allow it. *My* company frowns on getting too close. I have to keep my guard up. *They* tell us to keep our distance." Perhaps. But distance isn't really the issue in this context. It's comfort: comfort with yourself in leading two lives.

How could Dr. S operate as a vice president of a major hospital system, employing 4,000 people, and get away with being so comfortable with himself? *He* supervised people! *He* had responsibilities that would bury most of us, yet he never missed a beat at being himself. I asked the same question of myself at the time: How could I oversee a three-hospital rehabilitation program, with more than 200 employees, and survive as an integrated person? How could I be myself? *I* supervised people! *I* had significant responsibilities.

The answer was really quite simple: I had to stop taking myself so seriously. I had to realize that work is *what you do, not who you are.* Adopting a different approach to people at work was what created discomfort for me, so I decided to stop doing it. I was going to bring more of the real *me* to work.

Integration is not so much about getting close to people as it is getting close to yourself. As you will see in Section II, closeness is a delicate issue in a supervisory relationship, and gauging that distance is a constant challenge. In the current context, I'm talking about *you* bringing *yourself* to work. Don't leave the good stuff at home. Many times, I have seen young therapists put on airs the minute they get handed someone to supervise. They leave the nice person they were at home and take on this tough-guy persona when they approach their supervisory role. You do not need to do that: Be yourself and enjoy the benefits of moving fluidly between work and home.

Southwest Airlines was selected as the best Fortune 100 company to work for in 1997, and much of the credit is given to its CEO, Herb Kelleher. What is Herb's philosophy? "Work should be fun. We want a humanistic environment where people can be themselves." Simple advice from a successful executive.

Edifying

To edify is to build. If you cite dictionary definitions, you will also see, "to instruct" and "to build the mind of. . . ." Edification is on my list of management principles because it is a fundamental orientation that a supervisor or coach must bring to the game. You must go beyond merely instructing and building the clinical skills of your people to reach for higher things: the realms of self-esteem and personal momentum. This involves not just teaching, but looking for the inherent value in each person, in an effort to boost hope and inspire growth.

As therapists, we often frame "instructing" in practice terms, thinking that it only occurs when we are working with a patient, a family, or another professional who is learning a specific clinical skill. That is a given. That is the therapist part. Beyond this is the supervisor part, the role that brings growth to your supervisees in other areas associated with treatment, but not always mentioned, such as

- Teaching teamwork skills

- Helping with relationship building

- Dealing with campus politics

- Modeling conflict resolution

- Reinforcing mature behavior

- Helping with organizational skills

- Role-modeling positive feedback

- Demonstrating humility

When you embrace an edifying attitude with an individual or a team, you normally see a boost in energy. This profession attracts lifelong learners, and most of our members devour new information and positive feedback readily. A significant part of your job is to interpret the surrounding work world for your supervisees. That world might be the immediate team, an extended home-care staff, or a whole hospital. Through your ongoing advice, you build good corporate citizens if you conscientiously redirect behaviors for the betterment of all. If you fail to see your role as one of building effective work-community members, you shortchange your team and eventually yourself. At team or one-to-one meetings, you should occasionally hear yourself saying, "Now let's see what we learned from this experience," or "I see you learning, I see you growing." You are in a vital position to bring this edifying mentality to the industry.

A more obvious part of edifying *is* building clinical skills by helping to lay out a path for your supervisees. Continuing education is going to be a great challenge for our industry in the late 1990s, because training dollars are getting very, very tight. As recently as 1990, most competitive employers were offering from $1,000 to $2,000 per year for outside training—beginning the first year of employment. Now you are lucky if you can share in the cost of a $395 workshop on your own time. Nonetheless, broadening the clinical skills of assistants and aides is part of your role. Many companies are developing internal training divisions as a cost-saving measure, and that should help. In whatever way you can, you need to nurture clinical growth and take advantage of whatever opportunities avail themselves to you and your people. As you will see later, the goal-setting portion of the annual performance appraisal is an excellent time for planning training.

Ensuring Consistency
Consistency is perhaps the most treasured quality among friends and certainly among work associates. To be consistent is to be reliable; to be consistent and honest is to be trusted.

I once worked near one of the most inconsistent therapists I have ever met. She was usually late, arrived unprepared, was a horrific procrastinator, and served as a colossal source of excuses. A dedicated clinician at heart and champion of the elderly, she would work long into the night tending to her patients, but as a leader and supervisor, she was a disaster. She would hail the virtues of teamwork, only to violate most of the rules that good teamwork would dictate. She would act like a leader one day and like a 2-year-old the next. No one ever knew where she was, her notes were pitifully late, and she would often find that several people were overlapping on some of the projects she had assigned. How would you like to be an aide working for such a person? If you were the DON in her assigned nursing home, how long would *you* keep the contract?

The problem with inconsistency is that it breeds mistrust and resentment. If you are a therapist-supervisor making $45,000 a year for your 40 hours, a subordinate making $8–15 an hour has a right to expect some constancy from you. You are a *professional*.

Alcoholics create codependents in their families because of their erratic behavior. No one knows what kind of animal will walk through the front door at night, a drunk one or a sober one. If your moods, decisions, loyalties, instructions, and promptness are all over the map, you will see codependent behaviors emerge in your employees. If they like you, they will make excuses for a while. Then they will distance themselves. They will avoid you. They will talk about you behind your back. They will question your judgment. And when the first good job comes along, they will leave you.

I worked with a supply clerk once who was terribly herky-jerky in her moods, and the swings were all tied to a romantic relationship at home. At first, most of the office staff just passed it off by saying, "Oh, that's the way she is; love must be bad this week. . . ." Gradually, that phrase wore thin, and resentment set in. Orders were not processed, stocks began to wane, and people got angry. This woman was also a supervisor, and her staff felt that they could not approach her because of her testy moods. Her inconsistency in mood had become consistent, and the office was paying the price. Any worker—especially a supervisor—who is having personal difficulties must seek help outside of the office: friend, relative, pastor, counselor, therapist, anyone.

With all that is transpiring in the industry these days, consistency is a fine quality to bring to your team. You will be asked to deliver bad news such as mergers, buyouts, lost contracts, unit closedowns, layoffs, and reassignments—emotion-charged messages that come down from on high. If you have been consistent with your team over time, they can depend on you to be there, to explain what you can, and to carry their reactions back to management. The degree to which you embrace the remaining seven management values (particularly integrity and valuing teams) will determine how effective you are in the overall sense in delivering bad news, but I can promise you that consistency will go a long way in getting the job done.

Obviously, I take pride in being consistent. I work at it. It is not an inborn trait for anyone; however, it is essential for everyone.

Being Useful and Valued
Isn't it wonderful when you watch patients make progress and see that gleeful look of appreciation in their eyes? Isn't that why you came to work? Being useful is a great feeling.

Being useful and feeling valued are equally rewarding in a supervisory relationship. I have always regarded my supervisees as customers for whom I remove barriers to help bring success to their work. In fact, the most frequent quote my people have heard from me over the years is this: *If there weren't problems, there wouldn't be managers.* An occupational therapist (OT) friend of mine once said, "If you don't like to solve problems, you shouldn't be a therapist!" I would echo that—with a solid twist on the volume knob—when it comes to supervision. Problems are so much a part of management that you should make a conscious effort to accept them readily, not resentfully.

In the late 1980s, when I worked for a large Catholic hospital system, I participated in a leadership course that was mandatory for all managers. Among the many valuable morsels of management was a section titled, "Leader as Servant." At first I balked at this concept, because I failed to get the point. Why would I labor with all of this education and experience just to become someone else's servant? After several days of study and discussion, I got it, and it has stuck with me since. *We are all, in some fashion, in some place, servants to others.* If you tuck away your ego for a moment, pull yourself down a notch, and embrace the concept, it is much easier to accept those parts of the job that are often hard to swallow. You *serve* those assistants who need you to run through Medicare 101 again, because they need your help. You *serve* the tech who left the splint at the office and can't leave her home-care patient right now to go retrieve it, because there is no one else to perform that task. You *serve* the secretary who can't get her computer to boot the documentation program, because you have the skill and she needs you. You must learn to serve these people in the same way that you serve your patients and clients.

You are working in a profession of exceptionally bright people, and it is easy to get carried away with your own sense of self-importance. We forget, at times, that underneath it all, we are all just children whose shoes have grown larger, along with our responsibilities. Occasionally, we need to serve others and feel good about it. We need to be humble and helpful.

When I graduated from high school, I was voted "most helpful" by my classmates. At the time, I was actually embarrassed by the award, jealous of those who carried off the traditionally glamorous titles like, "most likely to succeed" or "most popular." I never mentioned *my* accomplishment to a soul for years. In fact, it wasn't until a couple of years ago when I realized what an honor it was to be valued so many years ago. Now, I'm immensely proud of it. Being helpful is a wonderful way to be perceived.

Perhaps I stress the importance of being valued because of my early years. I started working at the age of 9 as a paperboy and have essentially been working ever since. I slung horse manure, sorted eggs, dug weeds, stacked hay, painted fences, washed dishes, picked olives, and split stumps in high school, and in college, I mopped floors, delivered mail, pumped gas, sang rock 'n' roll, translated Spanish, filed medical records, took Fish and Game census, assembled skeletons, set up labs, glued furniture, painted houses, drove nails, and bounced at a teenage nightclub. That's a lot of trenches along the way, but it gave me an invaluable perspective on work life. It taught me to have the deepest respect for people at every level in every organization because of what they contribute. I learned that serving such people is a *privilege*, not a burden. I have supervised people with more education and income than I, as well as those with virtually no education who worked for minimum wage. It doesn't matter. Leader as servant is a viable philosophy, and I humbly suggest that you adopt it.

Sharing Love
If you have not picked up on it thus far, you might notice that love pervades much of my management philosophy. That might seem a bit odd in this bustling business world we endure, but love has served me over the years, both in my work as an employee and as an employer. It might well be the most powerful component in *your* set of management values, if you share it at every opportunity.

Tony Blair, the prime minister of England, eloquently quoted the *Bible* in his tribute to Princess Diana, in noting that "Love never fails." *Love never fails.* It takes a lot of love for a PT to go knuckle deep in the tunneled wound of an 80-year-old patient to prepare for a packing. It takes a lot of love for a COTA to absorb a painful slam in the forehead from a thrashing 9-year-old cerebral palsy kid who is getting splinted for a contracted wrist. Love is what gets us all past the choking stench of excrement from those patients who have lost their bowel and bladder control on our rehabilitation units. We might not be actively thinking about love at such times, but it's what gets us through the day, because love never fails.

As the survey clearly shows, love is why we got in this business. We love to put our hands on patients and love to see them thrive. I once watched a 15-year-old girl take her first step in a trauma recovery unit at the hospital and saw the tears flowing down every cheek around me. To say that the love in the room was almost palpable is an understatement. It was a once-in-a-lifetime experience for me. It was the ultimate sharing of love.

How much of that love do we bring to supervision? How much caring and understanding do we have left after a hard day of treatment? How much patience can we conjure up when an aide really screws up, leaving us legally exposed? How much love do we share when we have to do the dirty work—the really hard stuff—of management? How deep can we dig? How good can we be at leadership, in making sure that we preserve enough energy for our followers when they come to us with a problem?

Have you ever attended a going-away party for a particularly popular manager or supervisor? Ever see the gifts, the praise, the testimonials, the hugs, and the tears at the end? Think it was all about a paycheck? No way. It was about love, love given by someone who cared about her or his supervisees.

I once had to fire a very dear friend with whom I had built a volunteer-based drug treatment agency in central California. This woman was in her mid-40s and a total sweetheart, but she had not been able to keep pace with the steadfast rules of working with junkies. Among other things, she had been lending money to the clients for whom we were trying to find jobs, erasing the motivation we needed to get them to work (and enhancing their ability to purchase heroin on the street). Her kind nature—so effective in the earlier "drop-in" phase of the program—was now actually threatening the organization, because the funding source had gotten wind of the problem and was considering the withdrawal of support. I was faced with the biggest conflict of my early supervisory life. Instead of becoming the cold hard boss, distant and cool, I remained warm and close. I explained the situation in the most honest, direct terms I could muster and used my love for her and her work in acknowledging her contribution. It was painful for both of us, but not fatal to the relationship. We did this over wine and cheese. My employee remained a friend, and love did not fail either of us.

Another place where love shines through in supervision is where we must deal with situations that transcend the professional and enter the personal zone. Having to confront personality quirks, inappropriate dress, poor language, and even personal hygiene are situations I have faced. On one occasion, I managed a middle manager who smoked a pipe and had a terrible body odor problem. The combination was lethal, and other staff were issuing vociferous complaints. After several hints and casual comments, I was forced to sit down in a formal counseling session and put the job on the line: Either use deodorant or lose the job. Can you imagine? Because of BO? How uncomfortable is that? This was another person I respected and admired, and I *needed* his services. I reached deep to make that session work, letting him see that my love for him as a person was strong enough to cause me to be straight with him about something that was *very* uncomfortable for both of us. A bottle of Ban roll-on became a regular part of his office supplies from that day forward.

Love and respect are close cousins. When you face situations such as the ones I have just described, you can forget your sense of decency and just take the low road, as so many managers do. It is easier to let someone go by creating bogus excuses like budget restraints or differences in philosophy, I suppose, but in the long run you will feel shallower for having done it. You will lose love and respect for yourself, and the more often *that* happens, the less often you will be able to touch the lives of other people in an effective manner.

Beaming with Balance

In closing this section on management values, I want to stress the importance of balance. I have emphasized what many people would call the *soft side* of the scale in management values because they are the ones that most people forget in the mad dash to be successful. However, there is a very real, very sober *hard* side. Rehabilitation is a business, and for most of you, there is a profit to be made through your work. While you are attending to the ethics and personal virtues I've covered here, you must balance your work life with budgetary knowledge, computer skills, basic personnel law, training skills, and writing skills. You must prepare yourself for those employees who don't respond to warmth, kindness, and understanding, because they will try to take advantage of your kind nature. In the end, you will gain from being a benevolent boss; just remember that it's not *all* about feelings.

MORSELS

If you suffer from stage fright, here are a couple of useful tips I have learned and used over the years:

- Don't consume any type of caffeine within 4 hours of a presentation. Coffee, tea, and chocolate can hasten an unwanted anxiety attack.

- Try to avoid stress (particularly anger) on the day of a big presentation. There is a direct correlation between strong emotions and stage fright.

- If you can, arrive early at the site of the presentation and get familiar with the surroundings. This reduces alienation and fear.

- Try to meet some of the people in the audience before you get started. Make verbal and physical contact (shaking hands, etc.).

- Take charge of the situation when you begin—move people up, move yourself toward them, and so on—to make yourself more comfortable.

- Use media to help remove the focus from yourself, if that is helpful, but don't become overly dependent on overheads and slides.

- Use humor to lighten things up.

- Don't take yourself so seriously. People do not come to presentations wanting you to fail. If you carry critical parents in your mind, leave them at home; they probably wouldn't understand your talk anyway.

3
Relationship Management

A Look at What You'll Learn:

- Control, empowerment, and you: the pursuit of trust
- Why relationship management is a core function of the therapist-supervisor
- A new way to think about your customers
- How to think about organizational structure
- Dealing with friendships at work
- Perspectives on the "family" at work
- Dealing with dysfunctional employees
- The perils of middle management
- Growing into the supervisory role

The Empowerment Revolution

For the first 200 years of its existence, American business adopted a top-down, autocratic posture in its dealings with the work force. The all-knowing, all-seeing entrepreneur, *à la* Henry Ford and Howard Hughes, designed patriarchal work systems to exact his or her lofty dreams from the blood, sweat, and tears of loyal line workers. The unions arose in the early part of the twentieth century to combat the physical exploitation of these workers, but the basic philosophy of parentlike managers leading childlike workers remained. Until now.

A quiet revolution has been at work for the past decade. Business executives have begun to recognize that modern work is simply too harried and too complex to be carried out by robotic humanoids who leave their brains at home when they come to work. The multitude of daily decisions that must be made overwhelms an archaic system that demands higher approval from those who are the least familiar with the needs of the customer. In an ironic twist, we have come to realize that the real road to success is not at the top of the organization, but at the bottom. By giving line-level employees more decision-making power and asking them to take more ownership of the work, we enrich the organization where it counts most: where the work is actually performed. This is what is called *empowerment*.

Empowerment, like any good movement, has as many questions as answers: How can a corporate leader feel comfortable doling out responsibility to the lowest levels? Do you just suddenly change one day and turn everything upside down? Where do you start? How is empowerment manifested? What will the customers think?

Empowerment and Problem Solving

To exemplify the control-empowerment dilemma, let's take a look at two hypothetical private therapy companies attempting to respond to the same environmental threat. The problem is low census, the symptom is poor productivity, and the result is decreased revenues. Both companies are of medium size (±150 staff), and each has historically worked with a geriatric population.

Example 1: Top-Down Therapy, Inc.

After 3 months of successive decreases in productivity among licensed therapists, the CEO of Top-Down Therapy decides that he has had enough. He makes a few calls to colleagues to see if they have experienced similar reductions (they have), takes 2 days to make preparations, and calls a special meeting of all staff. Unlike the "general" staff meetings held by Top-Down, this one has no food or drink, no reports from the various departments, and no agenda or handouts. The CEO stands and waits for silence before giving a pile of handouts to his secretary for distribution to the staff. He then gives the following 2-minute speech:

> *Guys, I'm going to make this short and to the point. We have been losing revenue steadily over the past quarter, and it has to*

stop. Last month's productivity was below 50%, and that simply is not going to cut it. Today I am announcing that next week we will begin calling off any staff who can't prove to me that they can be at least 60% productive that day. We have far too many people sitting around, so we have no other choice. I will be meeting with the regionals and team leaders in a joint session to show them how to use the new form that is being passed out.

Also, beginning tomorrow morning, each therapist will be required to call the office to report his or her projected numbers for the day. Failure to call in will have serious repercussions.

I am very sorry about this, but things have changed considerably in the last year, and we must make sure that the company survives—for your sake as well as ours. You are extremely valuable to us, but we must get tough to help you keep your job. Things are tight in the industry right now, and virtually every company is having to do things like this.

Use the forms to figure your numbers, and keep them in a file, because we will be comparing your projections with the actual numbers at the end of each month.

Are there any questions?

Miraculously, there are no questions.

In the aftermath, there were several responses to these tactics on the part of staff. Several immediately gave notice and began working for registries while they sought full-time employment elsewhere. Several others took on contracts with home-care companies, arranged for afternoon visits, and made sure that they were sufficiently unproductive to warrant a daily call-off. Morale took an enormous plunge, office staff was reduced further, and therapists were deployed in two or more facilities with regularity. This angered the nursing home administrators, who were used to having "their" staff at hand, and contracts began to fall. The CEO sent out a hastily composed letter, assuring the administrators that all was well, but to no avail; the body language of his wilted and demoralized staff contradicted his words. Within 6 months, Top-Down had lost more than 40% of its business.

Example 2: TogetheRehab, Inc.
After several months of decreasing revenues, the CEO of TogetheRehab decided to get out of the office and do a bit of management by driving around (MBDA). She visited about half of the facilities staffed by TogetheRehab, touching base with administrators, DONs, and a sampling of her own staff. The process took 2 days. Three days later, at a regular management meeting, she shared her findings and threw the meeting open to brainstorming. In a 2-hour session, the management team decided to conduct a focus group in each building. A regional manager would be paired up with the team leader for that building, and a strengths, weaknesses, opportunities, and threats (SWOT) analysis would be done in an effort to build census, referrals, and cooperation with nursing staff. The meetings would last no longer than 2 hours, would be held over the lunch hour (11:30–1:30), and the results would be reported facility-by-facility at a general staff meeting to be held in 2 weeks. SWOT analysis is an inventory performed in an open forum by interested parties. If conducted with an honest, forthright approach, it can be very useful for planning or making changes.

At the general staff meeting, the CEO made the following announcement before entertaining SWOT input from the teams:

> *I want to thank each of you in advance for your contributions to the focus groups. I've spoken with several of you, and I have every confidence that your ideas are going to help us immensely. Between managed care, salary equivalency, and prospective payment, we have seen a drop in census that is hurting the bottom line. Therefore, as you know, we have opened all aspects of the company for discussion—everything from the benefits package to mileage reimbursement—to see*

what you think. I can promise you that no idea will be dismissed without careful consideration.

I must, in all honesty, issue a warning that some unpopular changes could also be implemented in the next few months. The management team would be doing you a disservice if we turned a blind eye to the low census and ignored the productivity problems. We are in this together, and I think we can survive without taking drastic measures.

I want to say one additional thing. If we are forced to begin calling off staff, I would like to know where each of you stands. If you have another income in the household and would welcome a reduction in hours, please let us know. If you can capture a few hours with another company to compensate for the reduction, we will work with you to help make that happen through creative scheduling. There has to be a happy medium in each situation, and we want to find that solution together.

The ensuing session was lively and useful. Several of the staff's ideas were implemented within the following 2 weeks, and productivity began to improve 6 weeks later. Because multiple-site deployment was one of the adopted solutions, the CEO hit the MBDA trail once again, this time explaining the changes in staffing to the administrative staffs of the nursing homes. Only one contract was lost as a result of the changes. Staff call-offs were eventually required, but the personalized approach limited losses to one therapist, whose financial situation demanded full-time pay. Also, to stay in touch with the feelings of the staff, the CEO created a monthly "chat session" for anyone interested in sharing her or his thoughts and feelings on an informal basis. This increased morale and confidence further, and TogetheRehab made it through its crisis.

If you truly believe in empowerment and don't just use it as a buzzword, you know that most of the answers to organizational problems lie with the staff. Top-down answers will work some of the time but will fail most of the time. If you pay the proper respect to the minds of your workers, you will harvest ideas and commitment as dividends.

You will thereby become empowered.

The Control-Empowerment Dilemma

An owner, president, or CEO has the responsibility of determining what an organization will produce and how it will carry out production and distribution. This includes developing designs that determine how much responsibility you will download to middle managers and the work force they direct. If the design is effective, employees will have what they need to perform the work (training and physical assets) as well as the ability to make decisions that please the customer (empowerment). If the design is flawed, the system will bog down, fall behind its competition, and eventually fail. While multilayered conglomerates might be more vulnerable, this bureaucratic thrombosis is not size dependent; companies of fewer than 100 employees fail every day because they simply cannot respond effectively at the line-staff level.

The key issue, particularly at the top, is trust. If an executive has invested his or her heart, soul, and savings in a company, how is he or she assured that the work is being done, that revenues are being collected, and that customers are being pleased without smothering the work force with control? On the other hand, how does the executive let loose enough to trust people who are half his or her age and four layers away from his or her title? Knowing that a negative contact with a single customer is said to contaminate a dozen other patrons, how does one legislate judgment? These are the questions that executives ask themselves in the wee hours of the night, every night. They add up to one of the greatest business challenges of the 1990s: finding the balance between control and empowerment.

There are no simple answers. There is no single formula for assuring the balance between control and empowerment at any level. As a therapist-supervisor, you have the same trust issues as executives, but in a more limited, localized, and focused fashion. Your teams are getting larger, the number of treatment locations is increasing, and you must trust work that you can no longer see or touch. How can *you* feel comfortable and confident? How can *you* be assured that the mission of the organization is being carried out by the assistants and aides under your supervision? How will *you* know if the customer is being well served?

In approaching these questions, I had a series of invigorating discussions with Karen Selley, OTR (then CEO of CMT), about the content of the workshop that would eventually lead to the writing of this book. Karen and I had long before agreed that the industry needed to gear up its supervisory skill for the era that was coming, and I credit her with pushing at the envelope to get our workshops started. As managers who had worked up through the ranks to executive positions ourselves, we had struggled with these control issues at several levels in our own careers. We wrangled with the concepts we wanted to cover in the workshops and kept coming back to *relationships* as the key focus for supervisors at the therapist level: the management of relationships, either directly or indirectly. True control can never be had, but *influence* through the management of work relationships could lead to greater success for therapist-supervisors, if we could just get the word out. If relationships could be strengthened, we would all be in better positions to solve the control-empowerment dilemma.

A New Customer

Rehabilitation is a business replete with relationships. Some are peer relationships, and many are customer relationships. In fact, defining the customers of rehabilitation is a study in and of itself. For the organization, the *primary* customer is the patient or client or student. As demonstrated in Figure 3-1, however, there are many intervening players that the organization works with who might be considered *secondary* customers: family members, nurses, physicians, teachers, and other allied health care workers. Without them, we lack

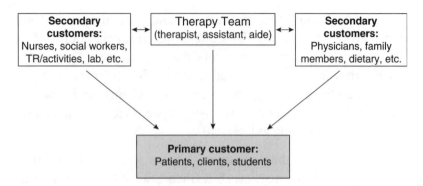

FIGURE 3-1. The primary and secondary customers of the therapy team. For the therapy team, the primary customers are the people directly served by the team: the clients in clinics, patients in hospitals or nursing homes, and students in schools. The secondary customers are those who help assure the delivery of such services, such as family members and other professionals on the extended team, such as therapeutic recreation (TR) specialists.

access and the necessary support system for successful outcomes with our primary customers.

I found it interesting in the results of the CMT survey that "developing professional relationships" and "the ability to get along with other professionals" ranked last or next to last as choices for what concerned students who were entering the profession. These were also the least-chosen items among experienced therapists, in terms of what challenged them or led to success in their work. As stated earlier, the top choices for both students and veterans related directly to patient-care issues, that is, the treatment of primary customers.

Are we truly so focused on treating the primary customer that we fail to prioritize these other relationships that are so vital to our success? Or are these data merely a reflection of an assumption on the part of therapists that professional relationships just "happen" because we are all professionals with common goals?

I think it is a little of both. Clearly, therapists are, above all else, oriented toward patient care. Given the choice, they will deprioritize just about anything else outside of actual treatment. They will assume that we are all in this together and that relationships with extended team members, such as nurses, will simply evolve over time. If there are bumps in the road, so what? They will come around. The nurses need us as much as we need them, so there is no need to take special measures with them. Here, at this juncture of the thought process, is where we need to do some work.

We *do* need to take special measures with "them." The management of these secondary relationships is one of the most significant activities carried out by the supervising therapist. The problem, however, is that these relationships aren't *your* relationships alone. As shown in Figure 3-2, you must now go beyond the primary paying customer described for the organization to define a second category for yourself: the people you supervise. You now have *two* primary customers. This is the duality facing therapists in the modern era. The assistant and aide relationships are the ones that you must manage most vigorously. As care extenders, they are now the front line of rehabilitation. More than ever, they will represent you. They are evolving ambassadors to all of the clinically related relationships that you need to maintain. How will you work *through* them to be sure that these relationships remain healthy? How will *you* balance your need to control them with your desire to empower them?

The answers are purely personal. I have struggled with these questions myself for years and continue to fluctuate as I work with new employees. Each supervisee brings a unique set of personal and professional traits, so a rote approach to developing trust is not possible. I must "learn" a person just as I would learn a new subject. I cannot truly control another person, but I can seriously influence what she or he does at work. So can you. You have at your disposal the same tools that I have: supervision, coaching, meetings, performance appraisals, merit increases, and promotions—structured opportunities to develop a relationship. You can stress the critical importance of the secondary relationships by making them a regular topic of the dialogue. You can help an aide or assistant prioritize a list

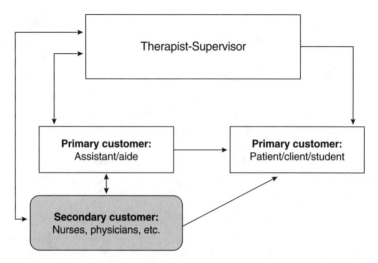

FIGURE 3-2. The customers of the therapist-supervisor. For the therapist-supervisor, an additional primary customer is added to the list: the assistant(s) and aide(s). This additional category creates a dual role for the therapist, who must divide her or his time between two related but different groups of individuals.

of key relationships that need to be nurtured, and visit that list at regular junctures. By so doing, you send a strong message about your attitude toward the value of extended team members—your secondary customers.

You can also serve as a role model for relationship building. If you listen well, provide support, follow up on commitments, and live out the management principles, your supervisees will know how to treat other professionals. You can be the leader-as-servant that they need to see. They will leave your presence feeling satisfied as human beings. Compare this with the angry employees who feel unheard, unloved, and unsupported by their supervisors. How eager will they be to reach out and touch someone?

Humility and the Secondary Customer
More than once I have heard hospital therapists lament, "I wish nursing would just leave us alone and let us do our work!" I suppose that this is

understandable frustration from those who are blocked from moving in a unilateral path forward, but it is not realistic. Who carries the treatment plan forward when a therapist exits? Nursing. Restorative. We need strong, viable relationships with our peer disciplines.

The human-to-human fabric that constitutes a relationship in rehabilitation varies from minute to minute, from place to place. We can carry a big stick in one setting, then drive 10 miles and be ignored in another. We are increasingly visitors on someone else's turf and are frequently forced to take direction from people of lesser education and training. I saw a lucrative nursing home contract go awry a couple of years ago, because a licensed practical nurse (LPN) had been elevated to the position of director of rehabilitation, and the therapy staff had a tough time accepting her authority. While it was true that the woman was fairly ignorant and misguided, her skill was not the issue. She had power and influence, and the therapy team did not. Once the LPN sensed that the physical therapy team demanded the upper hand in wound-care treatment, the end was in sight. Instead of backing off and strengthening the relationship, the physical therapy team charged forward, staking claim to sharp debridement (or else!), and the game was lost. The relationship had been poorly managed, and the contract was gone in less than 2 months.

Each rehabilitation setting has its own set of secondary customers. In the schools it could be a teacher or a counselor; in the hospitals, a physician or a social worker; and in the outpatient clinic, an HMO case manager. You and your subordinates will face dozens of situations like this in the next year alone, and you must reach deep to be humble, keeping in mind that it is the *primary* customer who will benefit from your patience in the long run. By combining the principles we have discussed with the skills yet to come, you will be able to manage these difficult relationships.

Organizational Structure: The Relationship of Company Relationships

Let's widen the lens and look at work relationships on a broader scale.

The structure of an organization is nothing more than the formal arrangement of its relationships. Vertical structure defines the hierarchy and lines of authority, and horizontal structure delineates the teams and how they relate to each other. I am a firm believer in organizational charts, because they offer a quick pictorial view of the north-south, east-west power lines of the company. Figure 3-3 reflects a typical organizational chart, with traditional terminology for the various levels.

Because I have worked with teams for so many years, I often talk of them in terms of the "triangles" they represent within the organization. Thus the width of a given team's triangle offers a comparative picture of the number of employees under the *direct* supervision of the leader. In organizational jargon, this is known as the *span of control*. Figure 3-4 presents two supervisory arrangements, depicted as triangles. Note that Team X has only two employees under a therapist (a narrow span of control), while Team Y has seven employees under a program manager (a wide span).

Much of the research in the service industry finds that a viable span of control ends at about six people; beyond that number, it is difficult to be an effective supervisor. My own experience corroborates these findings, although I have, at times, directly supervised as many as 12 people. It will be interesting to see what evolves in the next few years in the industry as things tighten down and therapists are asked to supervise five or six assistants or aides on top of (at least) a half-time caseload. Perhaps new models of efficiency for supervisor-therapists will be required.

The *span of jurisdiction* of the program manager for Team Y is extended to 17 employees when the assistants and aides are added, as shown in Figure 3-5. Unlike the span of control, the span of jurisdiction can be quite large, as long as the leader (i.e., the program manager in this example) delegates, supervises, and otherwise leads effectively. My prediction is that middle management positions such as program managers and coordinators will disappear over the next

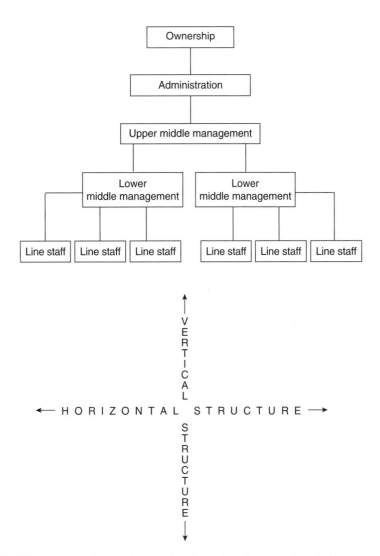

FIGURE 3-3. The typical organizational chart in rehabilitation settings has both vertical (top-to-bottom) and horizontal (lateral) components. Relationship development in both directions is of equal importance because of the interdependent nature of the work.

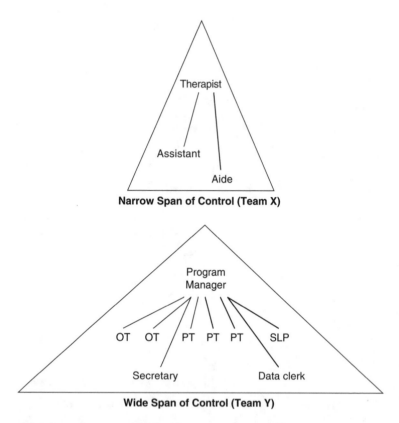

FIGURE 3-4. Span of control describes the breadth of supervisory responsibility assigned to an individual. It is generally assumed that the supervisor (the therapist or program manager in the examples shown) performs day-to-day supervision, coaching, and performance appraisal for the people under his or her span of control.

decade, with therapist-supervisors reporting directly to administrative personnel. As I mentioned earlier, this will, in turn, increase the autonomy at the therapist-supervisor level, not to mention the pressure to be effective as managers.

Our organizations are usually multilayered, and the titles of teams and individuals help distinguish the levels of authority and responsibility, while job descriptions lay down the work requirements and job duties. Figure 3-6 is an example of a typical hospital rehabilitation

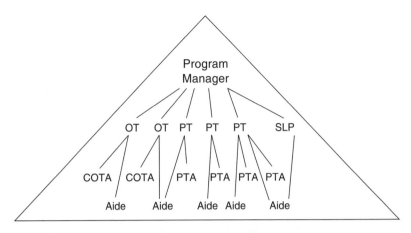

FIGURE 3-5. *Span of jurisdiction* is a term coined by the author to describe the number and types of positions under the indirect supervision of a supervisor, manager, or administrator. In this example, team Y is extended to include assistants and aides. For a program manager, the span could be a dozen or more; for an administrator, the number could be in the hundreds.

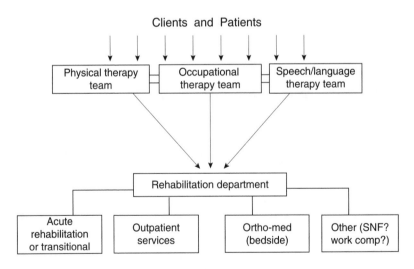

FIGURE 3-6. This organizational chart reflects the current situation in many hospitals, wherein the PT, OT, and SLP discipline teams serve the rehabilitation department in a number of potential settings. Gone are the days when a therapist could expect to retain a single assignment for a sustained period of time.

department, where subteams and extended teams are shown in an organizational chart. The emphasis here is on disciplines and deployment, illustrating the relationships between teams and departments.

Note that this chart is inverted, with the primary customers at the top, to make the point that it is the patients who should drive the work of this hospital. If you are computer literate, you can use word processing software to produce the squares, rectangles, and drawing lines you need to make nice organizational charts. Otherwise, do as I did for 20 years: Use a ruler and a pencil, and scratch out the diagrams you need to explain how you are organized.

A chart is supported by job descriptions. Job descriptions do not define relationships. People do. All a job description will ever do—in the best of circumstances—is describe what a person should *have* (training, credentials), what she or he should *know,* what she or he should *do,* with *whom* she or he should do it, and perhaps *where.* Sometimes, however, the job description fails to set expectations on work relationships. We should always see phrases like "develops working relationship with nursing" or " works effectively with team" or "acts as a team player" in our job descriptions to reinforce the importance of the human-to-human fabric.

Safe and Proper Distance: Friendship and Work

After all this talk about warmth, support, empathy, and love for your fellow employees, I am now going to tell you to find a safe and proper distance. What does that mean? Why would you want to do that?

For safety and credibility. Unfortunately, you have to be careful about the close friendships you develop with people at work. People notice who hangs with whom, how they act, and how it seems to affect the work relationship. When close friendships get intertwined in the vertical structure of an organization (e.g., supervisor with supervisee), it causes all kinds of problems: jealousies, accusations of brown-nosing, unfair biases, partial blindness, and so on. Credibility and effectiveness can be adversely affected.

I am not one to legislate friendships at work. I don't tell my people who they can hang with on their own time. However, I recognized early on that getting too cozy with colleagues can have a serious downside—particularly when the relationship is one of supervisor-supervisee. As a supervisor, you must always, *always* remember this: The close friend you make today might be the one you have to fire tomorrow. It goes with the territory.

Let me give you a living example. For 2 years (1995–1997), I supervised one of the top enterostomal therapy (ET) nurses in the country, a woman named Dorothy (Dot) Smith. We remain close professional associates. Besides being a terrific person, Dot is one of those rare individuals who is loved and respected by everyone she works with, without exception. She is a consummate professional, always with a good idea, always prepared, always on. She is the first to remember birthdays, the first to offer compliments and support, and the last to complain when things get tough. A truly wonderful person. But when Dot first started working with me, she said in her soft Louisiana drawl, "You gotta unnerstan' somethin' 'bout me. I'll love y'all at work, we'll have fun together 'n' do some great things here, but when I go home, I go home. I don't make close personal friendships while I'm workin' with people. Just ain't good policy. I like to keep 'em separate."

During our time together, I watched Dot dart and dodge through company politics, which were thick with strain, never once getting caught in the middle. She had probably the strongest relationships with peers among the staff in the home office, yet she consciously turned the key to "off" when she walked out the door. It had become a lifestyle choice for her. She was never caught in any professional snags because of a friendship.

This is a very delicate issue. People working in the same business are often attracted to each other as friends (or more), for obvious reasons. We share similar work interests. We have similar values. We enjoy exchanging war stories after work and taking aim at common enemies. It's relaxing and refreshing to have friends who really understand what you do, and why, and how. When I stressed being congruent with your work and home lives, I talked about the fluidity with which you can handle the various roles and how comforting it is when you attain a good balance. The only exception to that goal is this complication of supervisee friendships. If you get too close and lose your objectivity in the relationship, you not only compromise the role of supervisor with the friend, you erode the confidence of the remaining team members. They begin to question your motives, your judgment, your effectiveness as a leader. I saw this very thing happen with a manager who became blinded by a close, personal relationship with a supervisee, whose judgment she trusted without question. The problem was the supervisee manipulated the relationship for her own gains, and virtually everyone else in the immediate work environment became highly resentful. A manager whose integrity had never been questioned before was suddenly damaged in the eyes of her colleagues.

There is no universal rule for these situations. You, like Dot, must draw the lines that work for you and pay attention to the effects of your workplace friendships. It's just another angle—albeit a complex one—in the management of relationships.

The Organization as a Family: Asset or Liability?

For several years now, rehabilitation companies have marketed themselves as "families" in the pursuit of new employees. "Come Join the XXXCare Family" is often the lead pitch in journal display ads, with a list of mind-bending benefits to follow. The promise of warmth, security, and kinship is quite alluring, especially to new grads who are eager to regain the family they lost when they left home to go to college.

Is this a healthy approach in today's workplace? Is the promotion of company as family an asset or a liability? Are we increasing pro-

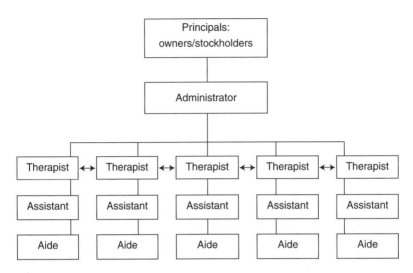

FIGURE 3-7. The flattened organization. As revenues decrease, the organizational model of the future could involve a single administrator supervising a cadre of therapists. This absence of support in the middle of the organization places additional pressure on the therapists to become effective managers of time and resources.

ductivity by creating a nonthreatening work environment or setting people up for disappointment with false promises?

Structurally, work organizations have been described by some as a series of vertical parent-child relationships, or *operational generations,* if you will, with each parent being someone else's child until you reach the top. In a company like the one shown in Figure 3-3, the lineage occupies five tiers. This would expand to seven tiers in a rehabilitation company, because assistants and aides would fall below the level of line staff, which would represent the therapist level.

While the degree of maternalism or paternalism within such a company is a philosophic issue, it is said that form follows structure. Thus a structure of this type lends itself more to a traditional family hierarchy than does the more horizontal, flattened design exemplified by Figure 3-7. This is not to say that the horizontal organization is by definition nonfamilial; it just reduces the obvious presence of hierarchy, creating a model that is more brother-sister than parent-child. Also, when middle management's presence is diminished, horizontal *inter*dependence is created, as shown by the bidirectional arrows between the therapists in Figure 3-7. I submit that this model, this reduction in the middle layers, will be the design of the future due to the financial constraints that are already being realized in the rehabilitation industry.

Viewing the work organization as a family has been a subject of discussion that goes far beyond rehabilitation. Peter Block, a principal architect of the empowerment movement, argues that a parent-child model is disempowering to the worker if it creates a false sense of security. By acting as a vocational caretaker and providing an abundance of benefits and annual pay increases, the benevolent company reduces an employee's drive to be responsible and to assume ownership, according to Block. It is also his contention that the inferred contract in the hiring arrangement is patriarchal in nature, such that business is simply carrying forward the same parent-child paradigm that has operated in primary and secondary education, the military, and the church for eons. In other words, if we perpetuate a parental model in our organizations, we don't allow our people to "grow up" into responsible, self-directed workers who share psychological ownership of the company.

Managers and therapists should not be thinking in terms of parenthood when they are supervising, for the reasons Block cited, plus a few others. For example, it has been fairly well established that adults unknowingly use the same language as their parents when placed in an authoritarian role, particularly when they are angry. If a company promotes a family model to the extent that it is acceptable to act like an angry parent when redirecting the work of an employee, I have a problem. Also, beyond creating a lax atmosphere, an overly secure environment can hasten dysfunctional behaviors on the part of employees who would otherwise toe the line in a more competitive work situation. We have all seen fellow staff members act like 2-year-olds at times, and it is doubtful that a more strict work system would tolerate such behavior.

In spite of these parent-child shortcomings, the family as an operational model for an organization has some utility. For example, the concept of loyalty to the clan begins at home, and most people will extend such attachments to the organization if it is so deserving. Loyalty, placed in the proper context, is a powerful motivator for most employees, one that should be cultivated in both directions: from employer to employee and vice versa. We cannot promise lifetime employment to anyone, and we should not expect undying dedication in return. However, for that period of time when we work in the same system, we can be brethren in the home of the work family. We can promote the same caring and loving that we bring to our primary customers, while reminding ourselves of the need to remain productive and profitable.

We often hear employees talk about the company family, and most people find that comforting. Where it exists functionally, I have heard therapists brag about the atmosphere, the support, and the social gatherings that feel so familylike. In other words, *it works well when it works*. Unfortunately, when companies undergo negative entropy and a hostile work environment emerges, the family moniker works very much against the cause; the leadership faces difficult decisions, and moving some of the kids out of the house is inevitable. Like friendships between supervisors and supervisees, familylike ties between companies and employees generate certain risks.

I use the family analogy quite often. It is useful in counseling a manager for being overly parental by taking too much responsibility in solving problems or for protecting an employee detrimentally. Most therapists can relate to the familiar language of such family dynamics. On the flip side, I see unhealthy dependency among supervisees, as well as sophomoric acting out in teams, and I am quick to point out that the family is weakened by such childlike behavior. You can make a case for sibling relationships (peer team members), cousins (peers on other teams), second cousins (extended team members, such as nurses), aunts and uncles (leaders of other teams), even grandparents (owners and other principals), if you really want to play with the organizational family metaphor.

In summary, there is no *right* answer about the promotion of a family atmosphere in our companies—there are only consequences. The consequences are negative if productivity and creativity are reduced in an environment made too warm and cozy, or by termination without fair and appropriate cautions along the way. The consequences are positive if the family and the parenting it promotes are genuine and realistic, such that all employees understand their roles as the children of the corporation.

Family of Origin and Health Care
The family of origin has much to do with the family at work.

More than once, I have heard that health care attracts more than its fair share of codependents. I am not sure about the accuracy of that statement, and I'm even less sure about codependency as a bona fide diagnosis. The concept of codependency emanated from the substance abuse treatment movement of the mid-1980s, when addiction specialists sought effective methods of dealing with the families of drug addicts and alcoholics. The theories about the antecedents to codependency were later expanded to include additional dysfunctions in the family of origin, such as physical and emotional abuse, extreme anger in a parent figure, and severe stress. The problem, as I see it, is that if you were to believe Bradshaw and Beattie (two of the more popular proponents of codependency), *everyone* would be labeled as codependent. Codependent behaviors include being overly dependent on others, enabling, being crisis oriented, acting persecuted, and being outwardly (as opposed to inwardly) motivated.

Codependency was never sufficiently embraced by the psychiatric community to be formally listed as a disorder. However, in my 20 years of working with damaged families, I did find that dysfunctional family behaviors learned early in life continue to show up at work. The at-work difficulties in our industry seem to come primarily from two sources: hyper-helpers and passive-aggressives (P-As).

If you've been in this business for awhile, you have witnessed the hyper-helper. This is the nurse or therapist or aide who can't do enough for the patient, the family, the peer, the boss, the janitor, the social worker, the guy on the street, and so on. This need often comes from years of making personal sacrifices to adjust to the antics of an out-of-control parent (or another significant relative), such that the person feels validated when she or he is in the helpful mode. Normally, we love hyper-helpers—particularly those working in aide positions. They do everything we ask, plus more. They will stay late, clean up the accidents, arrange all of our social events on their own time, and generally wear themselves out being helpful. They are workhorses.

Hyper-helper problems come in several forms. First, these people are often worn out from overdoing. They prioritize hands-on assistance and patient cheerleading, letting documentation go by the wayside. They overadvocate for the poor and oppressed, getting our teams in trouble with those who might have need to control the utilization of our services (e.g., managed care). Hyper-helpers often give the impression that no one else cares enough for the patient, so they become the chronic rescuer; this alienates other team members, distorts other patient-caretaker relationships, and just generally screws things up.

Probably the most subtle—yet deleterious—effect of hyper-helpers is their impact on the outcome of therapy. In most cases, the goal is to promote independence in the patient and appropriate support from the day-to-day caretaker. As a therapist, assistant, or aide, you need to resist the temptation to help with physical and mental challenges that could otherwise be performed by the patient or client. Although taught this important lesson in school, the hyper-helper blows right by the instruction, probably never even hearing it. When a hyper-helper is over-assisting with the eventual caretaker, the problem is further exacerbated, because that person (the certified nursing assistant [CNA] or family member) will most likely follow through with the same hyper-help that was role modeled in the instruction.

In my mind, the *passive-aggressive personality disorder* is one of the most destructive forces in any work environment. The classic definition for the term from the *Diagnostic and Statistical Manual of Mental Disorders* (4th ed.) (*DSM-IV*) is a "category for disorders of personality functioning that do not meet criteria for any specific Personality Disorder." In the extreme—the true psychiatric disorder—severe symptoms of depression, opposition, and aggression are observed. Most of our workers are not diagnosable as true P-As; they just demonstrate some annoying immature behaviors that *seem* psychiatric in nature.

P-A types tend to externalize blame for their failures, feeling jealous of those around them who are more successful. These are the folks who will give a warm, toothy smile when you're confronting them, and then blatantly bad-mouth you to four of your peers 10 minutes later. In other words, they are passive in your presence and aggressive toward you in your absence. When finally confronted, they will occasionally explode, but the normal tendency is to acquiesce. They tend to triangulate (and complicate) relationships through their avoidance, always choosing to take their problems to people other than those with whom they are having difficulty. In groups, this amounts to being aggressive toward one person by addressing the problem through someone else in the meeting; in my old psych days, we called this a "carom shot."

This is not a book on therapeutic intervention for the mentally ill. However, you do need to be aware of certain personality traits and how to deal with them. In the case of the hyper-helper, you need to curtail reinforcement for overachieving with patients and recognize the potential pathology. Do this carefully and over time, not with a sledgehammer in one session. The wronged hyper-helper is a highly resentful personality who can strike back—even violently—when feeling unappreciated. Most of these people spent years getting kudos for saving the world, and you are not going to change them overnight. Handle them with love and care. Most of all, avoid the temptation to take advantage. Don't work the hell out of them, and then cast them off once they burn out. I've seen that happen, and it's immoral.

The P-A types are much, much more difficult to deal with because of the nature of the neurosis. The dynamic is cyclic, because it is often impossible to get the person to talk to you about her or his behavior, and discussing it leads to more misdirected aggression. They are classic avoiders and effective gamers. Just last year I worked with a woman who would pile up relationship problems like bales of hay, only to dig deeply into her work (usually away from the office) to escape confrontation. This would go on for weeks, to the point where feelings were too polarized for anyone to talk to her about even the simplest of the problems she had caused them. Eventually an assault would come from some brave soul, she would nod and act agreeable, and say something like, "I didn't know you felt that way!" or "Why didn't people tell me I was causing problems?" or "Why do these things always come up when I'm gone?" Every response was directed toward someone else's behavior, never her own. A hug and a shrug, and she would be off, in search of more hay.

Dealing with a P-A (as we so lovingly call it) is as great a personality challenge as you will ever face as a supervisor. You will find yourself having to gear up just to have a casual conversation with someone for whom you have built up an intolerable amount of resentment. You have to reach deep for all the energy you have to be excessively direct and consistent; otherwise, you'll get buried.

I admit that I have had some difficulties in this area myself. My family was fairly dysfunctional, and I've had to work hard at being direct from day one as a manager. Perhaps that is why I understand the consequences so well: I've seen them played out too many times in my own private and professional relationships. However, I have learned that avoidance just doesn't cut it. As a supervisor and peer, when you have a problem with a coworker, you *must* go after solutions quickly and directly. If you are dealing with a chronic P-A, you must role model the proper behaviors, and stay after them to do the same. They might hate you, blame you, lambaste you, and then leave. Or they might listen, reflect, grow, change, and stay. Either way, your job will be easier and your company will be stronger for your honesty and directness.

On the positive side of family heritage, we often meet peers who were reared in homes rich with tradition for service to health care. It is not uncommon, for example, to meet therapists who are the heirs to the legacy of their parents and grandparents who served as physicians and nurses in another era. Having been raised in an atmosphere of dedication and sacrifice, they understand the lifestyle that attends the medically related profession. Also, I have found that people of this background tend to get along better with nurses and doctors because of their home-grown familiarity with medicine.

Parent Trapping

Parent trapping is a phrase I coined several years ago when trying to explain a specific phenomenon that occurs in middle management. It works vertically in an organization, usually downward from the parent level to the child level. This descending parent trap occurs when a middle manager (or a supervising therapist) is delivering an unpopular message from a higher level to the line staff beneath her or him on the organizational chart. Instead of owning part or all of the decision, minimizing the negative impact, and supporting management, the messenger extricates her- or himself and blames the "parents" for the lamentable directive. This gives the appearance of loyalty to the team, but has the effect of creating a common enemy of upper management. It is childish and destructive.

Such trapping can also happen in reverse, albeit less often, when a team requests the communication of negative feelings to the leadership. In this case, it is the *team* which gets trapped, because the team-trapping spokesperson divorces her- or himself from the message, acting as if anarchy reigns at the lower levels. She or he is merely the humble voice relaying the bad news, a victim of design.

Parent trapping is just plain bad politics. If you are going to be in any kind of leadership role—therapist-supervisor, middle manager, or administrator—you are going to have to learn to deliver decisions and directives effectively. This means asking enough questions to be sure that you understand the foundation of the decision, that is, the background music of the message. You might also ask exactly how the parents would like the message delivered to the kids. The last thing you want to do is walk into a team meeting and blurt out, "They did it again! Admin has decided to change all the forms. Don't ask *me* why, they just did. We'll have to start from scratch again. . . ."

With all of the changes going on in the industry, you will be facing these situations often, and the *delivery* of the news might become more important than the news itself. If you are forever coming on with the "here we go again" routine, you are going to demoralize your team and undercut your leaders. One year, when my management team had to reduce benefits to our employees for the second straight year in the face of tighter revenues, we faced several unpopular announcements. We orchestrated the sharing of the reductions, being careful to balance the losses with some good news about new business and new employees. We made certain that the spokespeople felt a universal buy-in before letting anyone meet with her or his team. It went quite smoothly, with minimal rebellion. It worked because we took the time to think about it and talk about it before moving ahead.

No doubt there will be times when you disagree with the message and don't want to deliver it. This is particularly true with new managers who still feel considerable loyalty to the rank and file and who feel prostituted by taking management's side. If this becomes a sustained dilemma for you, you must either reconsider your role in the organization or change companies. Not everyone in this business is ethical, and if you are being asked to do what goes against the grain on a regular basis, it's time to get out.

The Molting Process

The memory of my first day as a manager is as clear to me as a Rocky Mountain stream. I sat behind a gray metal desk and scanned a job description with my name on it. At the top were two words: executive director. *Executive? Me?* I had been student body *this* and class *that* since junior high, always involved in councils and committees and the other quasi-meaningless activities that schools tolerated, but never an *executive* anything. I felt like a 12-year-old grunt in a tuxedo four sizes too big. How would I fill up this enormous job title?

Like many of us who are prematurely handed the reins of leadership, I was not prepared for my first gig. I had no formal training, had read no books to speak of, and was flying by the seat of my pants. I was just there. Boom! One day a regular guy, the next day a supervisor. The only viable skill I had was group facilitation; T-groups and encounter sessions were the rage at the time, and I had gotten some good training, but that was about it.

Over the years, I've spoken with other ill-prepared managers who experienced similar feelings of inadequacy, and there seems to be some commonality as to how it goes. The growth of the not-so-ready manager is like the molting of an invertebrate animal: You grow your exoskeleton, slough it off, and grow it again. As you molt, you move along from child-like wonder to adultlike confidence, step by step, stage by stage.

The reason I like the metaphor of *molting* is because it connotes plateaus of growth, not continuous growth. Exoskeletons don't stretch; they are soft at first, are hardened, and then outgrown and left behind. Similarly, in management, your skills are often soft at first, then strengthened, and eventually cast off for stronger skills. On an emotional level, you *grow* into your new size (i.e., "flesh it out") as each new molt or plateau is attained. You make mistakes, do dumb things, hurt people, help people, have successes and failures, learn new tricks of the trade, and move on. It's fun to look back at the trail of slough in your past, saying to yourself, "I can't believe I used to do that!"

I find it instructive to connect the molting process with child development. We see the stages of child, adolescent, and adult in the behaviors and managerial practices of our leaders. And, as in child development, there are no clear boundaries in the growth process. You don't just land at the adolescent stage of leadership one day because you've survived some rite of passage; you take tiny steps, leap to new plateaus, molt a bit, flesh out the new level, take tiny steps, and molt again. Your confidence grows as you try out new skills and realize small successes.

Some day, after a particularly good meeting or performance appraisal session, in the privacy of your own mind, you might ask yourself: "Did I just molt?"

The concept of *relationship management* was treated separately in this book for several reasons. First, you don't want to look past this important activity in the rush to get your hands on the patient. Second, you must reprioritize your customers, in view of the changing work structure, and be certain that you are managing the *right* relationships. Third, you need to put your work relationships in the proper perspective, by paying attention to the ways in which friendship and professional kinship affect outcomes. And finally, you must develop a new identity in a new role, which is in essence the beginning of a new relationship with yourself as a supervisor. This is the philosophy of this book; the remaining chapters constitute the tools for carrying out that philosophy.

MORSELS

My ambivalence toward "family" organizations stems from experiences on both sides of the argument. I have been in organizations that were familylike but not parental, and personnel challenges were handled beautifully. Conversely, I have seen companies that practically promised a burial plot to their employees, only to become cold and distant when separation from employment became necessary. The difference, once again, lies in the expectations we create in the development of our work relationships. Consider the following:

- Love within a healthy family is unconditional and unending. The family emanated from the species' animal drive to survive. We rarely excommunicate family members for attitudinal problems or poor performance. When financial crises arise, we reduce spending, hunker down, distribute the workload, and survive as a family; rarely is anyone forced to leave.

- Love within a work organization is a completely different situation. The relationships, if they are made to feel familylike, should be framed with certain parameters. Love is not unconditional and unending. The organization has stakeholders who created it to produce a tangible outcome. Unfortunately, when certain provisos are not honored, a company member can be demoted or even removed from the "family."

- I would be the last to suggest that you withhold love and warmth from your employees; that would violate my own stated principles. However, I would be the first to say that you must cultivate a work milieu that affords you the room to maneuver effectively as a supervisor. This includes framing relationships conditionally. People must understand that your love for them at work cannot transcend their performance. For this reason, I prefer to use the term "familylike" over "family" to accurately describe the desirable situation.

II Performance!

An actress once asked in a Wendy's television ad, "Where's the beef?" In Part I, we took a brief look at the industry, a long look at you, a glimpse at organizations and relationships, and now we are here, in the trenches, on the job. This is the core stuff: Survival as a supervisor from hiring to firing. This *is* the beef.

I hope that you will approach this subject matter with the same fervor you bring to clinical studies, because this is the technical stuff that will get you through the day. The productivity demands on you and your charges are heading toward an all-time high, and you will find yourself beginning and ending your days with one big word stamped in your mind: performance!

4
Expectation Alignment: An Ongoing Process

A Look at What You'll Learn:

- Expectancy-valence theory and what motivates employees to work

- Boundary management and the war of two worlds

- What organizations expect of employees

- What employees expect of organizations

- How and when to seek expectation alignment

- Levels of alignment: company, supervisor, job

What Is Expectation Alignment?

Most of the theories on motivation and work performance were developed more than 20 years ago. Times change and so do people, but for the most part, there have been few new concepts in this area since the pioneers of social science did their work in the 1950s and 1960s. The one theory that I locked onto in school and held onto in practice is called *expectancy-valence* (E-V) theory (developed by Victor H. Vroom). In a nutshell, E-V theory assumes that people are motivated to work when they have the *expectancy* that the work environment will provide them with the outcomes they seek. *Valence* is the strength of the preference for those particular outcomes. In combination, expectancy and valence predict that motivation to work will be maximized when the employee agrees on expectations and rewards, and the employer provides work that allows the rewards to be realized. I refer to this as *expectation alignment*.

New employees enter the organization with a vast array of hopes and expectations based on the things they value. We normally think about salary and benefits first in this context, but those represent only the *extrinsic motivators*, that is, external outcomes that are a result of the work the individual performs. In a professionally driven industry such as rehabilitation, *intrinsic motivation* is equally if not more important, because therapists find considerable value in personal development, problem solving, and the ability to feel helpful. In the CMT survey, among the reasons for becoming a therapist, "income potential" ranked far behind "to help patients" and "interesting work." Other intrinsic motivators in rehabilitation include having good patient and peer relationships, contributing to the growth of the organization, and being a member of a team.

If E-V theory is valid, we must strive to design organizations that are primarily oriented toward meeting the intrinsic values of prospective employees. Then everything from hiring to supervising to evaluating performance is structured toward obtaining and maintaining alignment, assuring fit, and providing the proper rewards. It's just common sense with a theoretical backbone.

Let me give you an example from my own experience. I once hired a master's level psychotherapist to work for the substance abuse prevention and treatment company I was heading at the time. The salary was a little low for someone of her training and experience, but we were grant funded and had little leeway with salaries. Also, this woman was used to working in a clinic setting, and this job placed her in a local high school. She wasn't delighted about that, but seemed to understand the purpose of our approach. Finally, her expectation was that she would get to travel to exotic places and be trained in all of the new therapeutic techniques of the day. Because of the budget limitations (grant moneys for line items like training are often fixed in advance with few exceptions), we did most of our training in-house, in a manner similar to what is currently evolving in rehabilitation. For the entire 2 years of her employment with us, this counselor was unhappy. There was always the inference that we were cheap (We were! We had to be!), that her skills weren't being sufficiently tested in a school setting, and that we were shortchanging her on the training deal. I took the old-school approach and hired this woman almost solely on her credentials and experience, not on her *fit* for the organization or the job. She came in with a good attitude, but it eroded over time because we were not properly aligned. Her work was acceptable, but never stellar.

Expectation alignment should become a primary goal for you at all levels of supervision and management throughout your career. Also, as you will see later, it is an ongoing process. The example I just cited reflected an error in judgment on my part in the hiring decision. Expectancy alignment needs to happen every day, in many ways, at all levels. In working with your employees, you are continually asking yourself, "Are we using different paint on the same canvas? Are we harmonizing on the same song? Am I sharing enough of this game plan for us to win this match together?"

Boundary Management

At the level of a therapist-supervisor, you are a *boundary manager*. You are like the sentry watching the wall that separates two worlds: labor and management. Sure, you are technically "labor" yourself— as a therapist—but you are also the final level of management in the clinical hierarchy. You live in two worlds, and you interpret each of those worlds for the other. You walk a fine line.

As a boundary manager you must be keenly aware of the expectations of the company above as well as the needs of the workers below. The company (or organization or school) was here before the employee, and it pays your salary, so guess whose values you had best understand first! The company has a mission, a culture, a history, and a future that you will refer to when massaging the alignment of your employees. Some examples of important rehabilitation *company* expectations are shown in Table 4-1. Note that some of these expectations are vested in ethics, whereas others are more business oriented.

Imagine yourself as a therapist in a private, nonprofit, religiously based SNF, hiring your first assistant. You have just come from a large, publicly held therapy company that did business primarily in

Table 4-1. Company Expectations

Profitability
Quality of work
Quality of work life
Appearance of employees
Language
Demonstrated loyalty
Community image
Benevolence
Education and training
Reputation
Frugality
Teamwork
Customer service
Innovation
Market leadership

orthopedic outpatient clinics. Instead of having three people to supervise (two aides and one assistant), you will now have just one. As opposed to being responsible for some 20–25 *outpatients* per day, you and the assistant will have about 10–12 *inpatients* between you, with no aide for support. Which corporate values and expectations should you be focused on? Here are a few ideas:

- **Salary and benefits.** Every Assistant you ever hired at the clinic came in above $12 per hour; the SNF starts new grads at $8.50–9.00.

- **Productivity.** At the clinic, you were trained to do concurrent therapies and equipment rotations, and you had to keep three people constantly moving to meet the productivity requirements. At the SNF, they want high-quality relationships with patients and families and a slow, methodical approach.

- **Appearance.** At the SNF, there is a collared "rehab team" shirt (available in three colors), which can be worn with slacks or designer jeans and *white* tennis shoes. In the old days at the clinic, you could wear any jeans, shorts, and T-shirts, as long as they were clean. Most of the clientele was composed of weekend warriors and comp cases, and they didn't much care how you looked. Now the "clients" remember when Woodrow Wilson was their president, and they want you to be nice, well-dressed young women and men.

- **Language.** At the SNF, you are to nod to the nuns, speak in a soft, reverent tone, and never (ever) use profanity. Your prior job was loud and a little loose, with people goin' on, callin' you punk, or babe, or bud.

- **Documentation.** In your new life, you have rediscovered the ballpoint pen; nothing is automated. The only computer in the building is busy billing Medicare, and it was built in 1991. At the clinic, you just pointed and keystroked—nothing to it.

If you were hiring this assistant on your third day of work, you could be in a heap of trouble. The culture clash could be heard from here to Bangkok! As a boundary manager, you would be hard-pressed to bring the right person on board in the right way, because you don't yet know the alignment variables or the work culture; both are enormous issues in hiring.

Then there is *realignment.* There are times when companies are forced to take sharp turns in their businesses, causing managers to reinterpret the work world with *existing* staff. A great example of this can be seen in contract therapy companies. After years of contracting to provide services exclusively in nursing homes, some companies have diversified into assisted living centers (ALCs) and contracted home care. After diligently training the staff to be thorough in their evaluations and treatments—knowing that the Medicare reimbursement for OT and SLP was based on 15-minute units—the companies had to suddenly issue new orders: Maximize the effect of each visit in a minimal amount of time. Get in there and get out. In the 1998 version of home care, we get paid by the hour or by the visit, not by the

Table 4-2. Employee Expectations

Competitive salaries and benefits
Continuing education
Modern equipment
Compatible treatment philosophy
Strong support staff
Regular, useful supervision
Clinical competencies
Clinical ladders
Discipline integrity
Leadership
Clinical support (information)
Placement choices
Friendly atmosphere
Personal growth

unit. This is not only an awkward boundary situation for managers, it is an inconsistent message: Many of these companies had people working in nursing homes, ALCs, and private homes in the same day. Thus, a therapist is asked to maximize time (units) at a nursing home, only to drive 10 minutes to a home-care visit where time is to be kept at a minimum. Try keeping that one straight.

Earlier, I alluded to the hopes and expectations of new staff members coming into an organization. Obviously these feelings don't evaporate once you are hired, but they do change. They change because people learn, mature, get married, buy houses, move up, or just plain change. This makes realignment a maintenance issue, and we'll soon discuss maintenance skills. Table 4-2 lists some of the personal expectations that *employees* in rehabilitation might have of their company, either initially or later.

No matter which stage of alignment or realignment you are involved with at the time, this list (along with the company's list) offers some food for thought. The lists might not be complete, but they include most of the topics around which rehabilitation companies and therapists should seek alignment.

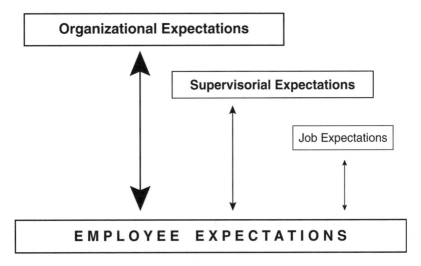

FIGURE 4-1. A cascade of expectations. The alignment of expectations occurs at several levels, as shown. The process of alignment for a new employee can take months, as he or she learns the norms, policies, and procedures at the three levels shown.

If we look at all of this from the perspective shown in Figure 4-1, we can see that there is actually a cascade of expectations (those of the company, the supervisor, and the specific job) that need to align with the one set of expectations (those of the employee). Each successive "umbrella" of expectations—from the organization to the supervisor to the specific job—is smaller, because the focus is narrower. Thus when misalignment occurs after an employee is already on board, we work from the smaller to the larger, trying to determine the following for the purpose of realignment:

- Is the misalignment reflective of a performance tendency, or is this person merely in the wrong job? Is she or he treating the wrong population? Is this the setting for her or him?

Or, jumping up one level:

- Is the misalignment reflective of a personality problem between this employee and this supervisor? Is an intervention

from a higher level manager in order? Would a transfer to
another supervisor help?

Or, jumping up one level:

- Is the misalignment reflective of a conflict with the organization's values and goals? Is this a person who will not make it
with this company, no matter where she or he is placed? Is termination or resignation in order?

Unfortunately, some supervisors feel that a nonperforming
employee is automatically a *poor* employee in the global sense and
that rousting him or her out of the company is the only answer. I
have helped accommodate transfers of jobs and supervisors for such
employees many times in my career, usually with good results.
Obviously the size of the organization has much to do with this strategy, because smallness limits the number of options available.

When Does Expectation Alignment Occur?

In Hiring
Hiring is mentioned first as an expectation alignment opportunity,
because it tops the list in terms of magnitude. *Hiring an employee is
the single most important alignment process you will embrace as a
supervisor; you will spend the rest of your work relationship with this
person continuing to realign in one way or another.* That is why a good
fit at the start is so important.

During Orientation
The process of alignment that was begun in hiring should continue
during orientation. We dig a little deeper, share a few tidbits about
each other and the company, and start creating loyalty. A written orientation checklist such as the one shown in Chapter 5 is helpful.

In Supervision and Meetings
The bulk of expectation alignment is done during supervision and in
team or staff meetings. With all that is going on in the industry,

external forces cause changes in the internal expectations almost daily. The earlier example of company diversification is a classic example of the need for dramatic realignment almost overnight.

During Performance Appraisals

As you will see in Chapter 7, the performance appraisal is a significant event for you and your employee(s), if it is treated with the proper time and respect. No matter how often it is applied, the work evaluation session affords both parties a *formal* opportunity to revisit alignment issues.

Within Corrective Action

"Corrective action" is merely a nice way of describing company reaction to individual work problems: poor performance, unacceptable attitude, strained relationships, or significant errors (of omission, judgment, or protocols). Although painful, these processes usually involve considerable discussion and opportunities for realignment and recommitment.

During Promotion or Demotion

Whether or not a formal interview is conducted during a promotion, there is usually the opportunity to digress a bit, bringing the respective dreams of employee and company together for comparison. The same is true with demotion, from a different perspective: When the movement is downward, the dreams seem more like nightmares.

During Exit Interviews

Alignment continues right down to the very end of the employment relationship. When an employee is departing, there is good reason to learn all that you can about her or his experience with you and your company. While such sessions are normally conducted by personnel (or human resources) staff, that isn't always the case—especially in small private practices of fewer than 15 employees. You might be asked to do the duty for an exiting supervisee of one of your peers or, perhaps, of an office staff member who is leaving. The knowledge you gain is valuable, if useful change comes from what is learned. Also, I have seen many rehabilitation employees leave and then return in a couple years, for whatever reason; the information in the exit interview—if given honestly and earnestly—can help pave the way for an even better work relationship the second time around.

It matters little whether you remember the specifics of E-V theory. It does matter that you seek expectation alignment between you, your company, and your supervisees. As you move through the next few chapters, keep that concept in the forefront of your mind; as a boundary manager, you are the medium through which the dialogue on expectations flows. You are the liaison between two cultures: corporate and worker.

MORSELS

Part of growing up as a manager is not fearing the misalignment of expectations with your employees. We cannot simply *will* people into wanting what they don't want or becoming what they are not destined to become. Just as love does not blossom between incompatible people, work does not flourish if the mutual goals are out of sync. To ask, at all junctures, "Are we together on this?" is more than courageous—it is smart. Better to have asked and parted than to have lingered with the fantasy that all is well when it is not.

5
Hiring: Finding the Fit

A Look at What You'll Learn:

- The parallels between hiring employees and treating patients
- Effective recruiting and hiring techniques
- How to screen and interview prospective candidates
- The amazing value of team interviews
- Orientation 101: How to initiate a new employee

Treatment as an Analogy

As I mentioned earlier, the hiring process is a critical opportunity to get off on the right foot with a new employee. And it is not just the final outcome (the hire) that is important, but the process itself. Learning occurs on both sides of the table, valuable experience is gained, and the value of the organization goes up a notch when a good fit is obtained. The lack of a successful hire—even after a lengthy recruitment and interview effort—should not be considered to be a failure; it is much, much better to have gone your separate ways than to have taken on an employee who is misaligned with you or the organization.

I took an informal poll of the participants at one of my workshops and was surprised by the results. I asked how many people in the audience had been involved in hiring in their careers, and only a dozen or so hands (out of 90 total hands, i.e., 45 therapists) went up. I thought virtually every company brought its therapists into the process, but I guess I was wrong. If this is indicative of the state of the industry, we need to make some changes. In my experience, the most successful companies are the ones that involve their teams in the hiring process. If it is done well, it is fun, and it is rewarding when you catch a big tuna.

Whether you have helped hire or not, you might enjoy this playful comparison between the traditional human resources (HR) hiring process and the traditional treatment episode (Tx). This comparison reflects the fact that you already have a feeling for hiring from your work in the treatment arena.

The Job Requisition = Request for Treatment Resources

HR: When you want to hire, you usually have to request the right to either create a new job or fill an existing one; this is accomplished by filling out a form or writing a memo to upper management.

Tx: In the clinical analogy, you are justifying the need for the training, location, equipment, or supplies to be able to treat patients or clients; a pro forma or spreadsheet showing the return on the investment for the expenditure could be in order.

Skills required: The ability to make your case; being able to accurately predict the revenues that will come from hiring or purchasing; the ability to write.

Recruitment = Marketing

HR: In the hiring process, you post, advertise, network, and otherwise get the word out that a position is available.

Tx: On the treatment side, you advertise, network, or just walk around (a process known as "trolling") to seek potential patients and clients.

Skills required: Clever, cryptic writing to describe a lot with a little, making the job or the treatment sound interesting; the ability to make and keep good contacts in the industry for networking purposes; the ability to accurately describe the job or the treatment available.

Seeking Resumes or Applications = A Request for Screening

HR: In hiring, you tell applicants to either send in resumes, fill out applications, or both.

Tx: In the clinical arena, you seek the right to look the patient over for possible evaluate-and-treat orders.

Skills required: Good judgment; good verbal skills; the ability to project an image of confidence and trustworthiness.

Resume Review/First Interview = Performing the Screen

HR: Not quite hands-on, just a feeling out, to see if you might want to dance; first interviews are usually done by just one person for efficiency purposes.

Tx: Similar concept, with an unpredictable hit rate.

Skills required: Knowledge of company HR policies/service reimbursement guidelines; good reading ability (resume/application/patient chart); good observation, interview, and listening skills; ability to gain the trust of the applicant/patient/client; customer service skills.

Narrowing to Finalist(s) = Requesting the Physician Order

HR: Justifying to yourself and others the decision to move forward with a candidate or candidates.

Tx: Clinically, convincing a doctor (or the nurse who calls the doctor) that a patient needs your treatment.

Skills required: Good judgment; ability to gain the confidence of superiors/physician/nurse; possibly good writing skills; customer service skills.

Final Interview = Doing the Evaluation

HR: Looking at the *whole* candidate, taking into account all of the factors that will result in a good outcome; aligning expectations with the candidate.

Tx: Looking at the *whole* patient to optimize the treatment episode.

Skills required: Solid judgment and assessment skills; good verbal skills; possibly group facilitation skills; teamwork orientation; documentation skills; customer service skills.

Job Orientation = Setting up the Treatment Plan
HR and Tx: Very similar activities in both worlds: discussing what will happen and how; setting short- and long-term goals; strengthening the relationship.

Skills required: Knowledge of company and job or of clinical discipline; ability to plan; ability to set realistic, measurable goals; verbal skills; writing skills; ability to teach; knowledge of proper documentation approach for the situation.

Performance Appraisal = Measuring the Attainment of Goals
Although this goes beyond hiring, let's play this comparison out.

HR: After the first period of work is completed by the employee, we measure progress and set new goals or modify existing ones. The employee could be discharged at this time, if such action is appropriate.

Tx: When the initial treatments are completed and rectification or rejustification is required, we grade the activity and act accordingly.

Skills required: Knowledge of HR/clinical policies and procedures; good judgment; assessment skills; good verbal and writing skills; knowledge of forms and proper documentation procedures; ability to plan and set goals.

Corrective Action = Amending the Treatment Plan
HR: On the HR side, this is the company's response to poor performance or aberrant behaviors.

Tx: For clinical, it can happen at any time, but usually during recertifications/rejustifications to either curtail, extend, or otherwise change the course of treatment.

Skills required: Knowledge of company/documentation policies and procedures; ability to confront people effectively; sensibility to seek HR consultation/managed care or case manager approval; excellent verbal and writing skills; ability to plan and reset goals.

Separation = Discharge
HR and Tx: Our comparison ends with the parting of the ways, either permanently or until the next time. Possessing good separation skills is useful in both situations, as well as in exit interviews (for employees) and customer service follow-ups (for clients/patients).

Skills required: Good customer service skills; ability to interview effectively; ability to reinforce accomplishments; knowledge of and ability to closely follow policies and procedures.

See how much you already know! In case it isn't obvious by this time, therapists, in general, are good at these HR-related tasks. You are good interviewers, have good judgment, know how to document, can observe and assess well, and understand customer service. Hiring is not a quantum leap at all.

Pre-Interview Tips
With the focus back strictly on hiring, let's talk about the interviewing process. A wild guess would say that I have probably reviewed more than 6,000 resumes and interviewed some 1,100–1,200 people in the past 3 decades, and hired 300 of them; the interview-to-hire ratio is roughly 4 to 1, which is fairly typical in white-collar work. Frankly, I don't have the time or inclination to wade through a bunch of unnecessary interviews, so I look those resumes and applications over carefully, do telephone screens, and make every attempt to narrow the list down to viable candidates. Here are a few tips you might find useful:

- *Be sure that the advertisement or posting is clear, accurate, and thorough.* For example, don't use a term like "assistant" when advertising for a COTA or PTA; you'll get applications for administrative assistants, office assistants, and every other kind of assistant imaginable. The same is true with technicians; the world is full of techs in virtually every field of work. You don't want engineering techs or computer techs or electrical techs applying for your rehabilitation jobs; it just causes everyone hassles. Also, it is a good idea to specify full-time or part-time, setting (hospital? clinic? long-term care?), and any special qualifications required (manual therapy skills, pediatric experience, dysphagia treatment skills, etc.). Finally, you might note that many companies list an address but no phone number. This eliminates the frivolous phone calls and puts you in the driver's seat; *you* review the materials mailed in, and *you* initiate the calls for the candidates you want to schedule. It is more expensive to be expansive in advertising, but you make the money back in time saved.

- *Read the application material carefully, at least twice.* By this time in your career, you realize the importance of written presentation from having applied for school and work positions yourself. I've seen tattered resumes, misspelled or misused words, unsigned cover letters, incorrect salutations, illegible handwritten letters and resumes, bright magenta stationery, you name it. All of those things make a poor impression, and few will get calls from me. I can accept a lack of understanding about the details of a position, but sloppiness is another matter—particularly in a licensed therapist. A sloppy applicant is most likely a sloppy documenter, and I/you don't need that!

- *Look for questionable employment patterns.* The two patterns I watch for most are the "job-jumpers" and "decreasing duration" types. Job-jumpers are those folks whose resumes look like the school record of a military brat: 6 months here, 1 year there, a gap, another 6 months, another gap, and so on. The decreasing duration resume appears less frequently, but it is also to be scrutinized carefully. These folks are usually older (and being seasoned myself, I'm sensitive to this bias), but their employment history is one of steadily decreasing tenure with each job: 10 years, then 5, 2, 2, 1, 6 months, and so on. I won't necessarily screen someone out for having this pattern, but I will certainly inquire as to the reasons. In fairness to the candidate, the problem could be traced to a spouse whose job required moving, family dynamics, or some other legitimate reason. It's okay to identify the pattern and ask for an explanation; it's not okay to ask about spouses, kids, health, or other personal questions that might violate federal or state employment practice laws. Be sure to consult your local HR expert on this and other employment-related laws before sticking your foot in it and getting sued.

• *Check a few references* before *the final interview.* This can be extremely helpful. After you have received permission and information to check references, make a few calls before the final interview. You will find that previous employers—if they are wise and informed—cannot verify much more than titles, dates of employment, and current status (meaning an "eligible or not eligible for rehire" note in the personnel file). In the case of the "not eligible" situation, you will most likely receive no details in the reference call. It will be your choice as to whether to proceed with that candidate, who can then decide how she or he wants to respond to your concerns. Always remember that the *employer* is not necessarily right in all separation-for-cause situations; sometimes it was the *fit* that didn't work, not the person. If I receive two "not eligibles" on the same candidate, however, I am finished; you rarely find a good employee who has failed with two other companies. Occasionally, you will find a reference who will chat awhile—particularly if the reference is good, and especially if it is outstanding. Just don't try to lure people into revealing negatives that they don't want to share; both of you could get in some serious (and expensive) trouble. Never, ever check a reference without permission from the candidate; some people are just checking you out, and a call from you to his or her current employer could raise many unwanted questions and problems.

Interviewing Tips

Frankly, I love to interview employment candidates. I enjoy trying to get people to relax, being creative with my questions, and matching the right person with the right job. I suppose I would tire of it if I did it every day.

Although I've made parallels here between employment interviewing and clinical interventions, only the required skills are similar; the dynamics can often be quite different. With a job candidate, *you* have something that person wants and the power to withhold it, whereas in the clinical situation, the customer is (usually) paying for the service, and the choice to be uncooperative is an option available to him or her. In both situations, however, I emphasize kindness and respect. Some candidates, just like some patients, are scared to death of you, and you must put them at ease to get what you want out of the interview. If you lord it over a candidate or patient, like some hotshot with a name tag, you'll never really know what was lost if you inadvertently shut him or her down.

Because my personal style is fairly casual, I prefer to interview people face-to-face, without a table between us. If a table is needed (for materials or writing), I try to make it a coffee table, to reduce the size and height of the barrier. This is a conscious maneuver to increase the openness for both of us. I want this candidate to know that I am confident enough now, in this interview, to be myself. I feel that this sends a subliminal message that I am probably that way all the time—someone you can approach, someone you can confide in. It works for me.

In the initial interview, I accomplish the basic goals of getting a physical look at the person (dress, demeanor, language style, responsiveness, degree of enthusiasm, etc.) while reviewing his or her training and work history. If I have a number of candidates, I might not delve into details—like clinical philosophy or specific skills—choosing to save that for the final interview. As a representative of my team, I have the responsibility of considering several variables in screening down to the finalists: personality, teamwork potential, attitude, and clinical background. I trust my instincts enough to know that I probably won't screen *out* a good candidate. If I only have a few people from which to choose, I will almost always leave two candidates for the final interview, to offer some choice. Leaving only one candidate from which to choose removes the comparison factor, thereby weakening the final interview.

My Favorite Five: Tangential Questions That Evoke Interesting Answers

Over the years, I have collected a few gems that go beyond the traditional "Will you review your work history?" or "Tell us about your strengths and weaknesses"–type questions. Those are important queries, and I use them regularly, but they do not always get at some of the underlying personality traits that I want to know about. Usually, I spread these (if I use all of them) across both interviews:

1. *"What would your biggest critic at work say about you?"* Next to asking them about their greatest weakness, this is probably the most difficult question for candidates to answer. Occasionally, there will be no answer forthcoming, and we move along. Most often, the silence is reflective of someone who (a) has never been asked anything remotely close to this question or (b) someone who has little awareness of her or his impact on other people. Perhaps the person doesn't seek feedback, or, if it is given, it is not acknowledged. I won't disregard a candidate who fails to answer, but I will ponder the implications. Humility is a valuable character trait in the human service business, and I want to employ people who are in touch with their deficiencies.

2. *"When do you feel most vulnerable?"* This is an "arrogance-seeking" missile. My biggest hope is that a candidate will think for a moment and say things like, "When I am behind and feel that I'm not doing a good job," or "When I have to speak in front of a group," or "When the DON calls me in for a lecture." These are healthy, normal exposures, reflecting a conscientious practitioner. My biggest concern is that I'll hear either, "I *never* feel vulnerable," or "All the time!" Oh, boy . . .

3. *"What gets you most excited at work?"* Many times this question will loosen up an otherwise tight interview. All the discussion about

school and work history and specific skills is aimed at the candidate, and the pressure brings out insecurities. Shift the focus to the work itself, and look out! I've seen soft, sedate candidates come alive at this question, suddenly bubbling with enthusiasm: "Oh, that's easy! The patients! I love the patients!" or "When I help position someone in a wheelchair who's been in pain for years, that is truly rewarding!" I even had one woman say she got most excited by "A nice, juicy wound!" Not a real turn-on for me, but clearly a reflection of her enthusiasm for the work.

4.   *"What situations tend to get you the most upset (at work)?"* The usual answers depict frustrations like, "A lack of follow-through after we get out," or "Not being able to get orders," or "Not having the right supplies." A few red-light responses are "People who don't agree with me," "Dumb nurses who don't know what they're talking about," or "Case managers who think they know more about the patient than I do." The first set of responses is acceptable because it demonstrates a genuine concern for good work and efficiency; also, they are generalized to the environment, without pinning the blame on one group or person. The latter set of unacceptable responses reflects an ego-based perspective in a negative tone, as well as a lack of sensitivity for teamwork (including a lack of sensitivity for the interviewer's perspective). I respect drive and professional integrity as much as the next person, but rehabilitation does not work alone. I will always take a modestly talented team player over a self-centered superstar.

5.   *"What other interests do you have, outside of work?"* This is virtually always a final interview question, near the end of the session. I like to see how well-rounded the person is, because balance tends to produce more happy, productive employees. There are no real flags on this one (short of, "Oh, I torture small animals on the weekends . . ."), although I don't like to hear that people spend *all* of their off-hours working somewhere else. With new grads, who are paying off student loans, it is fairly common and accepted; with vets, who stagger in exhausted on Monday morning, it gives me some pause.

Feel free to use my favorite five, or create variations of your own. My questions are not intended to provide some psychoanalytic manipulation, and neither should yours. However, because attitude is the basis for the majority of *for-cause* terminations, it is important to find ways to get beyond the usual "tell us what you can do" interrogation.

In closing this passage, I want to warn you about asking what I call "Duh?" questions. These are the obvious NCAA-approved, politically correct, Martha Stewart–endorsed, let me hear a big "YES! or NO!" questions. They are boring and unimaginative. Examples I have heard:

Q: Do you believe in teamwork?
A: Duh?

Q: Do you like to work with patients?
A: Duh?

Q: Are you a hard worker?
A: Duh?

I think you get the point.

Group Interviews: Time Well Invested

If you were going to adopt a teenager into a family of five, wouldn't you think it wise to have the rest of the family involved in the process? Can you imagine coming home one day and saying, "Hey guys, there's a young lady named Melissa upstairs in the back bedroom. She's your new sister, so please share your study desk, your toys, and the bathroom. You'll love her. She's nice!" Might as well burn the house down.

The group interview is probably the best investment of time you'll ever make as a hiring supervisor. Under most circumstances, I reserve group interviews for finals, but if a candidate is in town from afar, I will grab the opportunity and bring the team together quickly—especially if I sense a good match.

And getting the match is critical. Nothing maximizes the potential for fit like a team interview. In being able to ask their *own* questions and hear answers with their *own* ears, team members are more likely to accept a new team member once she or he is hired.

Moreover, they often ask questions from a perspective different from yours. They have their own agendas and their own views on how things are (or should be), and they will try to affect an interview to get at subtleties that you may never understand. Don't be afraid of that. If process is denied at the interviewing stage, it will come out somewhere else, perhaps destructively.

In 28 years of hiring, I have had but a single failure from a group interview. It happened when I overrode the recommendation of the team and hired a manager who lasted only 2 months. I tainted the chemistry of the group and paid for it.

It is a good idea to assemble the team a bit early, to assign roles (e.g., who will ask what, when), lay out ground rules, and answer any questions about the new position and the results of the first interview. New or inexperienced team members often remain silent during a team interview (out of shyness or feelings of inadequacy), so handing out jobs before the interview helps to legislate participation.

Be sure to begin a group interview slowly, with nonthreatening questions, such as "Tell us a little about yourself." Some people are very intimidated by groups, and you don't want to begin with questions that might unduly threaten them.

The payoffs for team interviews go far beyond a good hire. First, management is demonstrating its confidence in the line staff by asking them to help choose a new employee; this is an empowering act on the part of the company and is usually well received by the staff. Second, it is great experience. A taste of a management activity (asking questions, interpreting the work or the team to a candidate) is instructive and satisfying; it feels very adult to young staff members. Finally, I have often seen a team validate itself during team interviews. If they are particularly responsive to a candidate, a team will start selling itself, step-by-step, question-by-question. In fact, at times, the questions turn into statements: "This is a great group we have here!" or "You'll love it here, we really support each other." By the time we have reached that level of camaraderie, I just sit back and let things happen; the team has claimed the process as their own, and they are into it.

If you move on up to middle management, you will begin to notice other benefits from group interviews—particularly if they are being conducted by an intact, interdependent team. You will find that the process is educating *you* in a way that is not otherwise available. Even though you may have been meeting with this team weekly, they have grown in ways that you failed to notice. New leaders may have evolved without official knighting, and their prominence shows up during the interview. You may have lost control of this group and don't even know it. Although it might not *explode* in the midst of group interview, you will see the symptoms; most teams are wise enough not to upstage the boss in front of an outsider, but they will let you know in subtle ways.

One last note: In discussing opportunities for expectation alignment, I emphasized the hiring process. Be aware that the alignment isn't just between the new employee and company, team, or supervisor. It also occurs within the team, irrespective of whether *anyone* is actually hired. This is because the team hears you and its members discussing company history, the mission of the company, values, and so forth, with a prospective employee. It serves as a refresher course in company civics, a vicarious reminder of why this particular group of people is working for this particular company.

Orientation Done Well

Although it is not actually part of hiring, I wanted to emphasize the importance of providing a solid orientation for a new employee. While some organizations do a masterful job of orchestrating the first day, others fail miserably. More than once, I have reviewed exit interviews of employees leaving prematurely, only to find that they felt ill at ease throughout their employment because of having been short-changed with the *entrée* they received when they started. (More evidence as to the value of exit interviews, by the way.)

There is much to be oriented to in this business. The compensation-related details—salary confirmation, time sheets, pay periods, Social Security and tax forms, benefits package choices, cafeteria plans, and retirement issues—should be handled by those with technical expertise, like an HR representative. Don't mess with this stuff unless you really know what you are doing. Misinformation from you on tax exemptions, 401(k) deductions, medical and dental plan choices, or cafeteria plan calculations can result in a bad surprise on the first payday and a very angry employee. The same is true for the employee handbook, if you have one; company HR policies and employee rights are technical in nature, and an expert should be relating such information to new employees.

Finally, the basic health care entry requirements, such as vaccination verification, CPR training documentation, and licensure/certifications are normally done by departments other than rehabilitation itself.

Many (maybe even most) companies have an orientation checklist to guide supervisors through the maze of things to remember when showing the ropes to a new employee. If you have no guidelines, the following list of things to which a new employee needs to be oriented might prove helpful.

Personal and Professional Expectations

- **Appearance.** Appropriate clothing, including shoes; maybe length of hair, body piercing, and so on; impact on clientele (e.g., elderly are offended by certain types of clothing)

- **Language.** Degree of formality or informality of the work setting; relationship of language to clientele (e.g., the elderly, religious)

- **Norms.** Lunch and breaks; on-campus versus off-campus; sticking around to evaluate last-minute admissions, and so on

- **Disabilities/impairments.** Challenges to mobility, vision, hearing, and documentation capabilities; assistance or support needed

- **Work schedule.** Workday hours; overtime approval; weekend coverage expectations

- **Supervisory assignments.** If any; clear indication of responsibilities and authority; reminder of formal performance appraisal tasks

- **Safety.** Gait belts, maximum assists, transfer techniques, sterile technique, airborne pathogens, sharps, and so forth

The Immediate Team

- **Introductions/roles.** Personal introductions to new team; review of organizational relationships; who does what; who supervises whom (a list is helpful)

- **Meetings.** Frequency and purpose(s) of team meetings

- **Norms.** Social events, acknowledgments (e.g., birthdays), and so on

The Facility: Building, Hospital, School, Clinic

(*Note:* The emphasis here is on facilities away from corporate headquarters, where services must be dovetailed with the policies, procedures, and norms of another company's work system.)

- **Introduction to key players.** Critically important; facility staff *do not* like finding out about a new employee 6 days after they started; be sure that you are current on titles to avoid embarrassing yourself; remember the medical director and key doctors, if you can find them

- **Physical plant orientation.** Gyms, supply cabinets, wheelchair storage rooms, medical records office, etc. (A map helps.)

- **Mandatory/optional meetings.** General staff (including rehabilitation), Medicare/rehabilitation, department head, restraint reduction, special education, whatever; clarify what is mandatory

- **Facility norms.** Requirements regarding name tags, uniforms, shoes, stretching time, back support belts, and so on; expectations concerning social events, internal fund-raisers, daily prayer, charitable donations, and so forth

- **Equipment/supplies.** Orientation to equipment and special quirks/safety issues; review of relevant supplies (office versus clinical; who buys; issued to patient or building?); use of telephone, fax, and copy machines

- **Messages.** Telephone, fax, handwritten, e-mail, and postal mail; where do you get them, how do you send them?

The Company

- **Documentation instruction.** When, where, how, and what is required; how service is reimbursed, with which forms; training on computers and charting; transcription training (if any) and issue of pocket recorder

- **Continuing education.** How to request; approval process; procedures and norms (up-front cash versus reimbursement; shared expenses between company and employee, etc.)

- **Committees/task forces.** Names, purposes; how to volunteer; what to expect

- **Support services.** Secretarial, research, supply ordering; location of catalogues, library, videotaped instruction; professional support within the discipline; assistance with DME

- **Meetings.** General staff, discipline-only, quality assurance, and so on

- **Reimbursements.** Air travel, mileage, housing, and meal reimbursement for off-site services rendered

- **Name tag.** Nice to have one ready for the first day of work

The Job

- **Work assignment.** Title; type of patients/clients; clinical emphasis (neurologic? orthopedic?); formal job description is helpful

- **Location(s).** Mileage reimbursement; efficiencies in travel; buddying-up; salary equivalency guidelines in charging travel allowance, and so forth

- **Supervision.** Both received and given; multiple supervisors and matrix supervision strategies

- **Productivity.** *P*-word expectations for the assigned job. Does this vary for those who work across several settings because of travel time? Can the employee expect to be called off when the census is low?

- **Performance appraisal instrument.** This is important. Run through criteria and measurement system; explain any probationary-type reviews (e.g., 3-month application, if pertinent) and annual procedure; if self or peers are involved in process, explain

- **Initial goals.** Create three or four preliminary goals; this sets the stage for the supervisory relationship and gets the new employee rolling

The Supervisor

- **Style.** Review of how you like to interact with supervisees: Casual? Formal? Over the phone? In person? Regular feedback? Periodic? Direct? Do you give permission to disagree, to challenge?

- **Meetings.** One-to-one always? Supervision through team meetings? How often? Where?

- **Communication.** How you like to receive messages: Notes in your box? Memos to your e-mail? Faxes?

Off to a Great Start!

By now, you are saying to yourself, "What an exhausting process!" Yes, it is, when done well. But when you consider the time and pain involved in dealing with a poor hire, not to mention the cost of recruiting, orienting, and training a replacement, it looks like time and money well spent. And those are only the *obvious* costs. You can't measure the revenue never captured by an unproductive employee you hired through a quick and dirty process. You'll never be able to measure the damage to a team that was wrought by failing to include its members in the hiring of the wrong person. You might not ever realize that you lost a home-care contract because you hired a PTA who became so popular with the families that they never forgave you for terminating him for clinical incompetence. When I visit a high-performing therapy company, I can see how they became so successful: They built their organization the old-fashioned way—one employee at a time.

MORSELS

In a competitive business like rehabilitation, candidates will often judge the quality of a potential employer by the way the hiring process is conducted. The use of group interviews, enthusiastic participation by the team, and challenging questions combine to make a statement about the richness of your company. Strong, interesting people are attracted to strong, interesting organizations.

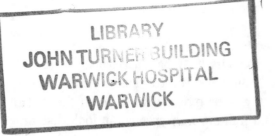

6
Supervision and Coaching: Keeping the Fit

A Look at What You'll Learn:

- How to supervise while promoting empowerment
- The difference between supervising and coaching
- How good coaching produces effective employees
- How to delegate with grace and effectiveness
- Tips to remember, transgressions to forget

After all the effort put forth to bring in well-matched employees, you certainly don't want to lose them. It's as if you have planted expensive seeds, and your job is to water, fertilize, and prune the seedlings toward harvest, hoping all the while that they are perennials. Supervision and coaching *are* much like tending plants: Give constant attention and love, and you will usually reap healthy crops. I hope to help you become an *organic* gardener, one who mulches and composts with honest feedback to keep the toxins out of the work soil.

For a single year, before returning to graduate school, I taught high school science, biology, and math—comfortable subjects that allowed me to stay one step ahead of my students in the curriculum guidebook. If there was one thing I learned during that long, yet enriching year, it was that although I had a teaching credential, I couldn't be expected to know *everything*. I began to use two phrases that have helped me as a teacher, parent, and manager over the years: "I don't know, but I can help you find out . . ." and "Where have you looked for the answer?"

As a supervisor, you might have a tendency to put undue pressure on yourself to be the expert and instant problem solver. This is understandable and quite common; after all, you are being paid more than your supervisees (usually), and they look up to you for answers. If you are a "pleaser" by orientation, you want to be helpful, and you see this function as a major part of the supervisory responsibility. Conversely, you might be a therapist-supervisor who takes an alternate route: You focus on your own clinical work and help your assistants and aides when you can find the time. You see the supervisory role as something of a nuisance that pulls you away from the patients.

Vision: Not Always So Super

To discuss this issue of responsiveness more closely, let's look at two extremes: overdoing and underdoing.

The Near-Sighted Know-It-All

Leaders who adopt nearsightedness as a modus operandi feel that they must be the end-all and be-all of answers and solutions for their charges. They smother people with support and extinguish the joy of discovery. Empowerment is born of self-generated efforts to learn, solve problems, and assume ownership for one's work, and it must be honored and revered. The overzealous supervisor, just like the doting parent, steals a precious opportunity for empowerment from the worker each time she or he overresponds and takes charge of the solution. By leaping buildings in a single bound, the SUPERvisor, in effect, strips the thrill of victory from those who are not yet close to the jaws of defeat. Rarely do I see an adult who truly *enjoys* having everything spoon-fed by an elder; it defies human curiosity and crushes the spirit.

The Myopic STUPORvisor

At the opposite pole sits the unresponsive supervisor. Although suffering from myopia, this supervisor actually needs a prescription for bifocals. It seems as though tending to two worlds (treatment and supervision) is too much, so only one of the planets gets attention. Not being able to see beyond her or his own work, this person is not particularly approachable, fails to follow through on requests for information, and is of little value to the team as a leader. In fact, he or she is usually seen only when there is a problem. The unspoken message is, "Don't bother me . . . unless you absolutely have to!" Simply stated, STUPORvisors like this should not be managing anyone's work. They let problems smolder, and breed resentment among other employees. If you go back to the core values of management, you will recall *that being useful and valued* was on the list. Nothing irritates employees more than people who hide behind their titles and do not carry their own weight. Being responsive and helping to solve problems conscientiously is part of the weight of being a good supervisor.

I guess if I had to make a choice, I would opt for a know-it-all SUPERvisor over an unresponsive STUPORvisor; better to have a doting parent than a deadbeat do-nothing.

Think Before You Help

To be an effective supervisor and coach, you should act as a leader, sounding board, consultant, supporter, and general resource for your employees in a manner that promotes thought and growth. There are times when you should attempt to answer questions on the spot—in crises or when simple procedures need to be explained—because that is helpful and appropriate. However, when more complex issues arise (such as clinical questions requiring research or interpersonal hassles requiring courage and confrontation), you might balk a bit and involve the employee in finding the solution. This takes sensitivity and judgment, because it is delicate.

In a family model, this philosophy amounts to effective parents raising inquiring minds; parents cannot learn for their kids, and they should not want to. For example, my 12-year-old son, Devin, has always been an excellent speller. From the first grade on, he could review his weekly list once and pretty well nail every word on it. Earlier this year, however, he began asking me how to spell simple words, because he found it easier than using the dictionary or the computer. Yesterday it was the word *unusual* and last week it was *situation*. At first I bought into this tendency to find the easy way out, because it made me feel wise and important to be such an instant resource. Eventually, however, I began to realize that I was fostering poor learning habits. Devin was getting lazy with his spelling, and I was buying right into it. Now I always respond with, "Try sounding it out," or "Why don't *you* take a crack at it first?" This not only keeps him sharp, it prevents a needless dependence on me (and in the future, other "experts").

Once again, finding the balance between competing forces is the answer. You *need* to be responsive, you *want* to promote growth, but you *must* somehow reconcile the two in order to be effective.

Supervision Versus Coaching

In the world of rehabilitation management, you hear the word *supervision* almost daily. You rarely hear the word *coaching*—it's just not part of the normal vernacular. Perhaps it should be. Consider the following distinctions in the definitions from *Webster's*:

- *Supervision, n;* to oversee or direct (work, workers, a project, etc.); to superintend.

- *Coach, v.t.;* to instruct (a person) in a subject, or to prepare (a person) for an examination by private instruction; to train and instruct.

Supervision, at least according to the dictionary interpretation, is more coordinative in nature, involving work, projects, and the worker(s). Coaching is more educative and more individualized, moving the employee through a step-by-step process. Also, supervision tends to focus more on the past (what has happened, how did it happen, who was involved, etc.), whereas coaching is future oriented (what will you do, how will you do it, with whom, and when?).

Supervision: The Operational Necessity

In the job descriptions of our industry, we use terms like "oversee" and "direct" to outline the responsibilities and establish the authority of the manager over her or his staff. While "provides training" might also be included on the list, the supervisory duties are normally operationally oriented to include such things as "assigning caseloads, assuring productivity, approving hours, ensuring team-work," and the like. These are valuable and necessary functions, to be sure, and traditional in the framing of a supervisor's job. Much of the supervision in a team-based environment like ours is a fostering of interdependence and, therefore, somewhat global.

Mentoring is another familiar management-related term. The term derives from the literary character Mentor, who was a friend and counselor to Odysseus. The formal definition of a mentor is "a wise and faithful counselor." In our field, mentoring has been chan-neled toward the development of clinical skills, usually in a one-to-one relationship. It is a close cousin to coaching and could be used interchangeably.

Coaching: Development of the Individual

Coaching, in comparison to supervision, is more personally focused on the development of skills in the individual. It is also more inti-mate in its application, requiring a give-and-take that feels more peerlike than normal supervision. In coaching, we attempt to break a work task down into manageable steps, much like we would in treating someone with a physical or mental disability. Some of our people—especially the wallflowers who coast along under a strictly team-based supervisory model—will flourish under personal coach-ing, if given the chance.

I like the concept of coaching in rehabilitation because it is familiar territory for most of us who have grown up around sports. When we coach an athletic *team*, which is more of a supervisory function, we are dealing with the overall game plan: teamwork, posi-tion assignments, assessing the competition, game strategy, substitu-tions, working the clock, and so on. The coaching of an *individual* athlete precedes the game plan, of course, because it involves devel-oping the skills that will contribute to the overall mosaic on game day. It is at this level, I believe, where great coaches are distinguished from merely good coaches. Virtually all successful athletes—at the professional and Olympic competition levels—have personal coaches, testimony to the value of the this type of teaching.

When we coach an athlete, we assess physical skill, mental tenacity, ability to enhance a team effort, and competitive performance. We coax, cheer, motivate, direct, redirect, argue, judge, criticize, encourage, acknowledge, and reward. We *coach* that forward to lay the pass gently into the outstretched arms of a breakaway guard by practicing the drill over and over. We *coach* wide receivers to run the precise, predictable routes toward the quarterback's targeted spot in the corner. We *coach* the shortstop to deliver a soft, catchable throw to second base, for the chance at a successful double play.

In carrying the coaching concept into the clinical realm, I try to remind therapists to allocate time for thinking. With the hands-on work that we do, we often find ourselves charging through the day accomplishing tasks without a lot of forethought. Personal planning and focused *thinking* are not skills that come automatically, so a little coaching on conscious anticipation can be quite worthwhile. For example, we can *coach* a PT to think beyond a stage III wound to correcting the poor bed positioning that caused the pressure ulcer in the first place. We can *coach* an OT on how to make her own splints when managed care won't pay for the expensive ones. We can *coach* an SLP to handle two feedings at once because breakfast lasts only 45 minutes. We can also coach our supervisees through presentations, conflicts, proposals, or anything else they might fear by asking questions and helping them to find their own answers. Coaching is an active process of vigilance, repeated observations, and trials.

Once Again: Seek Balance

In making choices on how to spend your management time, you should try to balance supervision and coaching. Tend to the operational details, but do not forget the individual developmental needs. As a therapist-supervisor, you cannot assume that your staff arrives on the job trained and disciplined. You must observe and coach, coach and observe.

One determinant of how much emphasis you put on supervision or coaching is the makeup of the team beneath you. Strong collective clinical skills within the team might mean less need for coaching in that area on your part. However, interpersonal deficits among team members might mean more emphasis on supervision and team building. The needs will fluctuate several times in the same year as the team grows and changes, and people go and come; you will need to weigh the balance as you go along.

And then there is *you*, with your own traits. Depending on *your* strengths and interests, you might have a tendency to swing one way or the other on this supervision-coaching pendulum. If you tend to be a shy person, not wanting to work in groups, you might lean toward coaching, because it tends to be performed individually.

Last year I worked with a management team that included two women of opposite dispositions on this issue. One, an SLP, was intrigued with the supervisory aspects of her position, so she buried herself in the technical team duties at the expense of the individuals. She loved creating documentation manuals, work schedules, and new treatment programs, so that is what she did, spending little time developing her employees. It was her perception that *coordination* was the job. Across the table from her sat a PT whose orientation was almost *exclusively* toward clinical skill development. She was a master trainer who loved to roll up her sleeves and get her hands dirty, but her team—in the operational sense—was a disaster. Schedules were goofed up, vacation coverage was not arranged, meetings were missed or mis-scheduled, and productivity waned because people were always off being trained. This therapist was highly respected as a coach, yet disdained as a supervisor. These two women, both good therapists, strike another strong case for finding balance.

Coach as Chameleon
Effective coaching, like effective supervising, requires putting on a different face at times. Often, people respond to the same approach in different ways. To be effective, you must become a student of human

behavior. You must *read* people well. You must adjust your style for each individual to maximize the benefit of your expertise in a teaching/coaching situation. The SLP I mentioned above was ineffective as a coach because she never looked up; she talked her way through feedback, gave rote responses as to how experienced she was, and rolled onto the next treatment manual. I once parted ways with another clinician who had the unfortunate habit of treating all of her employees with the same basic approach. "No nonsense!" She would bark at them. "I've shown you how to do it, now go do it!" Frankly, I found her quite refreshing in this era of coddling and pleading, but I also realized that this approach simply didn't work for some of her people. I would hear that she was "out of control" or "too aggressive" in exit interviews and through the grapevine. Throughout our time together, I implored her to apply the same wonderful assessment skills with her supervisees that she reserved for her patients. I encouraged her to soften a bit with the high performers (the folks who would buy her the moon at the mere wrinkle of her brow) and get even tougher with the resisters and the gamers. She was a superb clinician and a growing coach.

Coaching at Altitude

Having worked at all levels with a variety of volunteers, paraprofessionals, and professionals, it is my observation that *coaching* has not been as prevalent at the higher levels of management. The assumption, I suppose, is that baccalaureate-or-higher–level people are trained and educated and not in need of coaching. I don't *agree* with that assumption, I just observe it. If you move up the line into formal management positions, you should try to pursue coaching for yourself from those who work above you at a higher level. If that is not available, you might consider a *personal* coach. With the advent of the Internet, e-mail, and personal 800 numbers, personal coaching is becoming an affordable alternative to expensive workshops and consulting.

Hands-On, Yes; Feet-On, No!

Compared with the world at large, we work in sophisticated environments. Our people are, for the most part, well educated and achievement oriented. You don't graduate from the professional schools these days without some smarts and a solid work ethic. Yet I still run into an occasional supervisor who clamps on to a supervisee like a cowboy on a bucking bronco. Hands-on supervision and coaching is one thing, but *feet-on* is another.

If you think back to the management values, you will recall several terms that relate to respect: the *Golden Rule, integrity, honesty, goodness.* When new employees come aboard, I approach them with these principles in mind and assume that they are decent, dedicated people who want to get the job done. I assess their skills, align expectations, and set up the supervision and coaching regimen that appears to be required. As we move along, I recalibrate and either increase or decrease the amount of coaching that is needed. I trust this process.

The bronco riders I mentioned do just the opposite. They fear the worst, assume nothing, and overdo it. They disempower and discourage valuable employees. When is the last time you heard anyone say, "Boy, I really like the way he runs herd on me!"? Admittedly, there are times when the cowboy approach is necessary, but only in response to identified deficiencies in such things as time management, judgment, clinical skills, customer service, or interpersonal relationships. Riding herd should never be your initial approach.

Delegating with Grace

Learning how to delegate effectively is almost an art form. So many of us, when faced with too many tasks, think, "Oh, I'd rather just do it myself," or "By the time I teach someone to do it, I could have done it myself twice." Sound familiar? I have personally used those excuses myself for years. My own self-sufficiency can become my worst enemy. When we discuss self-management, you will see that delegation is a skill that requires discipline. It needs to become a habit.

Habit or not, there are a number of simple steps to be considered for delegation to be done effectively. Delegation is a technique of supervision, with all of the dynamics that go along with managing a project done by someone else. Here are a few thoughts:

- *Always be courteous and considerate when handing off a task or project.* Don't be unkind and let your self-importance blind you to the reality of those working beneath you. Even though you have the power to demand help, don't. *Ask* for cooperation and assistance. *Ask* about the status of the person's workload. *Ask* how his or her day is going. The respect you show will be repaid many times over.

- *Communicate the results you want.* If you need a written report, ask for one. If you expect this person to present results to a group, tell him or her now. If you want someone to look into travel arrangements, or tickets, or supplies, or equipment—but don't want a purchase to be made—be clear.

- *Anticipate problems.* Helpful hints are greatly appreciated—little tidbits like, "That nurse can be cranky in the morning, so just nod and go along with her until she calls in the order; she's really a sweetheart beneath that tough exterior," or "You have to spread the terminals on the cord of that frying pan before you plug it in; otherwise you'll sit there all day waiting for the paraffin to melt." These are the things that people appreciate and remember.

- *Clarify the level of authority and responsibility.* Can the delegatee make critical decisions? Is this committee just a recommending body, or do they have the power to act? How much responsibility are you actually willing to give away?

- *Set deadlines and discuss duration.* Whether you are delegating to a person or a committee, people deserve to know the time restrictions under which they are working. This is an extension of mutual respect. Also, the duration of the assignment is important: Is this a permanent role? Is this a committee (usually medium- to long-term) or is it a task force (usually short-term)?

- *Provide adequate resources.* Remember how annoying it was when your dad asked you to mow the lawn and then drove off without unlocking the tool shed? Most projects need resources beyond the human, so it is important to discuss what is available. In the clerical arena, this might mean copying, printing, transparencies, travel arrangements (flights, car rentals), or special arrangements (flowers, meals, microphones, etc.), depending on what is to be done. In the clinical arena, it could be supplies, equipment rental, audiovisual setups, training materials, vehicles, you name it. Don't fail to let people know what they have to work with.

• *Schedule a brief "check-in" session on large projects.* When assigning a large, complex task, arrange for a formal meeting midway through the project. This can help prevent delays for the shy or overly self-sufficient employee who will fail to ask for help (or clarification) on an assignment.

• *Assure wrap-up and feedback.* Obviously, we don't do a formal "wrap-up" for a small task like cleaning up after a meeting, but we should provide acknowledgment. Because of time constraints, we are forced to ask people to do some pretty awful things (clean up feces on the mat, blood on the parallel bars, etc.), and a little pat on the back goes a long way. With bigger projects, a thorough review of successes and challenges is extremely useful. Feedback is not only educational, it is endearing—people like the attention after having worked hard. Feedback on failure(s) is particularly critical, and it should happen as soon as possible, following completion of the project. It is a terrible disservice to withhold constructive feedback.

The Unforgivable Five: Terrible Transgressions Among Therapist-Supervisors

By now, you have a fairly good idea of where I am coming from in terms of values, style, and priorities. Here are a few of my management pet peeves: the five most terrible transgressions among therapist-supervisors.

Number 1: Failing to Follow Through

When I worked in the hospital system a few years ago, I used to lunch in the cafeteria once or twice a week, because the food was actually very good. Invariably, I would overhear a CNA or a housekeeper or a maintenance worker going on about a superior. It usually went something like this: "They never do nothin'. They just sit up there and collect the big money! We ask for this, they promise that, but nothin' ever gets done. Someday I'm gonna be a supervisor and sit on my butt for a livin'. "

This example might not be from therapy, but the underlying feelings transcend all lines of work. The fact is, people expect performance from their supervisors. And nothing reeks of poor performance more than the lack of follow-through. It gets noticed. You can't hide. An individual or team depends on you for some kind of resource or decision, and you simply cannot fail to come through. Simple as that.

If you do fail to follow through on a promise, for crying out loud, own it! No one is infallible. To err occasionally is human, and people will accept that, as long as it doesn't become a chronic lifestyle. If follow-through is a problem for you, be sure to review the section on time management.

Number 2: Delegating Inappropriate Tasks
This one has both political and legal implications. There are tasks that should be legitimately expected of aides to help the assistants and therapists be more efficient and productive: setting up charts, ambulating patients, cleaning mats and equipment, documenting, copying, filing, calibrating equipment, the usual stuff. However, that does not include performing nonprofessional duties, such as the personal shopping requested by the SLP mentioned in an earlier chapter. Moreover, when a therapist or assistant gets the reputation of continually handing off *all* the crap work to someone else, the word gets around, and both aides and assistants will avoid working under that therapist. I have heard aides whisper things like, "You never notice her (a PT) with dirty pants; she hasn't been on her knees to help treat a patient for 10 years!" The habit of *over*delegating is not illegal per se; it's just impolite and unwise, creates an unnecessary alienation, and dampens team spirit.

Speaking of the legal front, you must remain acutely aware of what your practice allows in terms of delegation. Having an assistant perform an evaluation or allowing a PT aide to perform sharp debridement of a wound is clearly contraindicated, and you risk a number of legal and financial exposures with that type of inappropriate delegation.

Number 3: Violating Confidentiality

If you want to see the trust and respect from your team members go south in a hurry, just make a habit of breaching their confidentiality. Highly interdependent communications such as supervision, coaching, and performance appraisal are much more effective in a milieu of trust between the participants. Supervisees often confide in their superiors to gain advice and expertise (if not catharsis), and such courage should be revered. Stressors such as domestic struggles, family illness, private lifestyles, or personal depression are often shared during these sessions, and the supervisor has an enormous obligation to protect such information. The following statements, made by therapists I have worked with personally, are some typical examples of unacceptable violations:

- "You can't trust *anything* she does in the morning; she's an alcoholic, and she comes in hung over. I talked to her about it just last week."

- "Well, you know he's on the verge of a divorce at home. He actually broke down and cried in my office last week. I think he's going to quit."

- "Oh, don't let her bother you. She got a lousy performance appraisal from me, and she's feeling bitchy."

- "She finally admitted to me that she was gay just yesterday."

Information is power. When you move into a supervisory role, you must raise your personal integrity a notch and become a responsible adult. No more junior high antics, no more playing with people's lives; as a supervisor, you are the banker in the commerce of relationships below you, and you cannot afford to spend trust frivolously. Corrupt supervisors who wield personal information as some kind of weapon have no business being in a leadership role.

Personal information is often pursued. Some people will seek you out and attempt to lure you into revealing personal information about others, because they find it titillating. I worked with an employee who had a nasty habit of aligning herself with you against what she perceived to be common enemies to extract confidential information (which she would, in turn, use against you). "You know," she once lamented, "that guy is a terrible CEO. I hear that half of his staff is ready to quit. Didn't he tell you that he was in over his head?" If I got sucked into this game and said something simple and seemingly innocent, like, "Yeah, he did say something like that," or even "Yeah, I know what you mean," I would breach confidentiality and be set up for a fall. The entire office was well aware of this manipulative scheme, and everyone avoided personal conversations with this highly destructive woman.

Some of us have problems with polite refusals in such situations. Because violations of confidentiality are so lethal, I want to leave you with a few handy phrases to use when faced with inappropriate inquiries about personal or professional information:

- "Oh, I wouldn't feel comfortable talking about that. . . ."
- "Well, you know that's really confidential information. . . ."
- "I can't really get into that. That's personal stuff. . . ."
- "I'm a little surprised that you are asking. You wouldn't want me to share that kind of information about you, would you?"

It's easy to reflect on the Golden Rule right now, isn't it?

Number 4: Being Chronically Indecisive

A distant cousin of "failure to follow through" is indecisiveness. Sometimes a lack of follow-through is due to the inability to decide, sometimes not. Over time, a team will usually figure it out, because indecision on the part of the supervisor is fairly obvious. And annoying.

How many times in your life have you heard, "I would rather that he make a poor decision than none at all!"? I am not sure I agree with that philosophy, because snap decisions can also be hurtful; I want thoughtful, careful supervisors out there on the floor. However, this attitude on the part of supervisees is reflective of the frustration they feel in the face of chronic indecisiveness.

Obviously, when decisions are delayed (or *never* made at all), progress is stalled, and people begin to lose faith in management. At the end stage, they stop asking altogether and either end run or leave.

If you *repeatedly* hear yourself saying, "I'll get back to you," or "Let's put that off for awhile," or "I'll have to ask about that one," you might have a problem with making decisions.

When I am working with indecisive managers, I ask to them to consider the following questions:

1. Do you understand your job?

2. Have you been given enough authority to make such decisions?

3. Are the questions or requests appropriate?

4. Is this the right position for you?

Making decisions with due diligence is a great challenge facing the new supervisor. If you are fresh out of the blocks, don't be too hard on yourself. Weigh the variables carefully, and *ask* for time if you need it; that will be respected by your team. Ask for *help* if you need it; that should be provided by *your* manager. As you grow, the decisions should come easier; if they don't, back up 10 spaces and reread the four questions above.

Number 5: Failing to Respect Others
Saved for last, this is the big momma. All four of the previous goofs contain elements of this transgression. Disrespect erodes relation-

ships like rust on a nail. *If you fail to understand the fundamental value of being respectful to your coworkers—no matter their station in the work force—you will ultimately fail as a supervisor-coach.* Here are a few scenarios—including the reactions of those disrespected—to reinforce that point.

- A therapist continually fails to schedule meetings with her team on the rehabilitation unit, choosing instead to assemble spontaneous gatherings whenever she feels like it. *Team reaction: "Boy, our time certainly isn't worth a squat! We aren't even worthy of advance notice."*

- A rehabilitation services manager decides to reward his team for reaching 70% productivity 5 weeks in a row in their assigned nursing home. He holds a lunchtime party in the rehabilitation room, which is walled by windows in the main hallway of the facility. *Facility staff reaction: "Thanks for inviting us to the party, bud; it's not like we had anything to do with the census that is giving you your units!"*

- A contract therapy company administrator repeatedly invites subordinates into his office for discussions and talks over his shoulder to them while scanning the Internet, never once making eye contact. *Staff reaction: "What a colossal jerk!"*

- A veteran OT supervises a bright young COTA who is ripe with fresh approaches to the work. Three times in 1 month, she takes those ideas and claims them as her own at the company management meeting. *COTA's reaction: "Thanks, babe; let's see how creative I get with you next month! First option at a new assignment, and I'm gone!"*

Disrespect for people's time, their contributions, their ideas—it all adds up. When you read of great women and men of the world, people who have really made a difference, you will often hear the word "respect" in the same sentence. This is because most successful people possess an integrated view of the world; they know that their self-respect is only as strong as their respect for others.

The Fabulous Five: Tried Tricks of the Trade

These are a few of my personal favorites, little acts that often fail to make the big management books. Take a look and see if you find some elements of your style on this list.

Number 1: Complimenting Work Well Done

If a few more supervisors would just take the time to acknowledge good work, our industry would be much stronger. A simple pat on the back or squeeze on the shoulder goes such a long way with so many people. "Good job," or "Well done," or "I really appreciate that . . ." is all it takes. Although I think that I have always been a supportive manager, I must credit my old mentor, Dr. S (who is actually younger than I), for role-modeling the power of giving compliments. Talk about a hands-on manager! The good doctor would flow through the office, onto the hospital floors, into administration, through the cafeteria, and back to the office, issuing little thank yous, acknowledgments, and remembrances for this and that, always with his hand extended in one way or another. He always gave credit where credit was due. He knew that his success was primarily due to the work of the people under his jurisdiction. You could literally watch the pride and loyalty grow before your very eyes.

If you come from the school that thinks, "People are *paid* to work, so I don't need to compliment them," you had better go back to class. *Everyone* gets paid, but not everyone gets acknowledgment. Just pay attention to this small detail. Notice I didn't say *minor* detail, because it is not minor at all.

Number 2: Celebrating Victories and Acting Out on Holidays

At times, work life can become quite stale. We motor along for weeks, doing our respective things, with few peaks and valleys to mark the time. As a supervisor, you are in a position to create topography in the landscape. You help set goals, so why not set celebrations? When I worked in the grant economy, I always appreciated the tradition of having happy hours when a large proposal finally hit the post office. We didn't even know if we would get the money, but because the writing of a grant was such an awesome undertaking, we had a party to send off our lofty tome to Washington. It helped to keep people pumped. Think of all the things you could do! How about being told by the SNF administrator that you have to complete 30 screens in 2 days? When you and your team finish, party down! Or how about that OT who just got her hand therapist certification? A cause to celebrate.

We have to find more ways to make work fun. Especially now, when things are getting tight in the industry. If you work a 40-hour week, you spend 35.714% of your awake time per week at work (assuming you sleep 8 hours per day), and work is best done in a holistic environment. I love it when staff dress up for Halloween or wear goofy ties and shirts for St. Patrick's Day. It brings managers down a notch, and the patients love seeing their therapists in holiday clothing. In schools, the kids go nuts when the teachers dress up, so why not the therapists?

The old expression, "You can make a difference!" definitely applies here. You have a team and you have some power. Use it.

Number 3: Dream-Making
I once heard an inspirational speaker named Dan Miller talk about his life as a polio "success story." As a teenager, Dan contracted the virus just before the nationwide vaccination program ended the epidemic that plagued America in the 1940s and 1950s. With his entire right side essentially paralyzed, Dan overcame formidable odds to become a successful physical education teacher, school principal, pilot, and guitarist. He gives credit to those wonderful people who, along the way, encouraged him to take risks and meet challenges; he calls them *dream-makers*. Dan places his wife Judy high on that list, because her cheerleading helped urge him to new heights many times.

Dream-makers are those people who listen to your story or watch your work and say, "Yes, you can do this. Keep trying!" They are the ones who make that extra phone call or look for that special book that will inspire you. They are the ultimate edifiers who help you to believe in yourself. I have had a few myself, and I'm sure that you have your own list.

I once worked with a PT who had a particular knack for dream-making. On two separate occasions, she went far beyond the norms to help get employees into PT school, simply because she believed in them. One was her baby-sitter, and the other was a rehabilitation aide. For the baby-sitter, my friend flew 2,000 miles just to talk the school into accepting her as a student, which they did, and now the woman is one of the most respected neurologic PTs in Colorado. The aide received reference letters, financial support, and summer work while she trained in Australia. In 1996, she returned to work as a PT in the company she once served as an aide.

The components of dream-making are not magical. Just good listening, imagination, support, and a little extra effort. And the rewards will stay with you and your "dreamees" for a lifetime.

Number 4: Aiming at the Middle
There will be many times in your career as a therapist or manager when you are asked to deal with a consumer complaint. The "consumer" might be a patient, a family member, a charge nurse, another therapist, or a physician, and the complaint could, of course, be just about anything. "Aiming at the middle" refers to entering the scene on neutral ground, honestly intending to understand the situation without bias. It's much more difficult than it sounds. As a member of the clan, the primordial response would be to defend your own. But what if your teammate has erred? How effective will you be, with both guns blazing?

Conversely, what if you consistently assume that the customer is always right and begin maligning your own staff before you have both sides of the story? Last year, I had a situation involving a wheel-chair seat cushion. A nurse had called our therapist in to take issue with "the fact" that our assistant had incorrectly installed a 4-inch cushion upside down, causing a pressure ulcer to develop overnight. The first thing out of the therapist's mouth was, "She [the assistant] should *never* have done that!" It turned out that *housekeeping* had inadvertently flipped the cushion while cleaning the chair the previous afternoon, and the assistant had nothing to do with it. Needless to say, once the word got back, the relationship between the therapist and the assistant was seriously tainted.

A few neutral-tone phrases are helpful in depolarizing such charged situations. They are useful on both sides of the fence, no matter the source of the complaint (i.e., your staff or a nonstaff person):

- "I'm sorry this happened. You are obviously very upset."

- "Okay. Let me see if I understand exactly what happened. You feel that . . ."

- "I don't know, but I'll look into this immediately. Can I get back to you this afternoon?"

- "This is pretty complicated. Let's sit down and break it down, step by step."

Notice that the *middle* is the center of several things here. The speaker is expressing concern about the situation and an acknowledgment of the complainant's feelings, but not (yet) an apology; she or he doesn't know if an apology is in order at this point. Also, no one is implicated in these responses: neither the complainant nor the employee. Some kind of follow-through is promised in the third statement, but not necessarily a solution; there might not *be* a solution forthcoming. Finally, the last response brings activity to the problem immediately by initiating a discussion, which is halfway between a silent shrug and a shouting match.

I admire customer service experts who can aim at the target and hit the middle with a satisfactory resolution. It is a skill I continue to work on.

Number 5: Cultivating Creativity

The final feature of the Fabulous Five is truly a wonderful quality for a leader to have. Whether it occurs in a team meeting, in individual supervision, or across the lunch table, the ability to stimulate the ideas of others—without becoming threatened by them—is an admirable leadership trait. Creativity is a vulnerable plant with delicate flowers that can blossom or wilt according to the quality of the surrounding air. Strong leaders who cultivate the fresh air of creative freedom in their doings amplify their effect many times over by bringing out the best in those around them. With simple acts of encouragement ("That's really interesting—tell me more!" or "What a great idea!" or "You guys are *so* creative!") and the ability to follow through, the leader-cultivator will always reap the sweetest fruit.

Final Thoughts for the Supervisor-Coach

Arrogance is a particularly aggravating quality in a person. When it is combined with ignorance, it is dangerous. To be ignorant is to be human: No one knows everything. It is said that Thomas Jefferson was the last American to have mastered the available knowledge of his day, yet even Tom was learning anew until the day of his death. He could not have created the Declaration of Independence, a true masterpiece, without respecting the collective knowledge of his peers.

To be arrogant is to be closed: New methods rarely get through, and when they do, they are barely recognized. The arrogant are so taken with their own sense of self-importance, righteousness, and focus that they are deaf to the ideas of others and threatened by the skills they lack personally.

Arrogance and ignorance in the same person is a lethal combination. When vested in a leader, it is virtually intolerable because of the amplification across other people's work. It stifles creativity, hastens resentment, and kills the satisfaction of otherwise meaningful work. It makes meetings boring and ineffective, taints self-image, and chases valuable talent from the rank and file.

If you want to be a successful supervisor-coach, you must recognize your areas of ignorance and tend to them. You cannot possibly know everything; in fact, you don't *want* to know everything. If your knowledge is so great that there is little room for the thoughts of others, the creative energy of your staff will dissipate in a thin, barely audible vapor. Being an effective leader means being humble enough to know when you are in over your head. Seek advice from both above and below you, and use it wisely.

The most obvious flaw of the ignorant-arrogant personality is its feeding of itself. The very person who is ignorant is too arrogant to realize it, too self-centered to listen, and too pig-headed to change. These people maneuver to eradicate the source by firing, transferring, or otherwise removing threatening personnel who might expose their shortcomings. These are logical, predictable survival techniques for the exposed individual, but deep, possibly fatal wounds for a team.

Take inventory. If your meetings are flat and draggy, dominated by you and your agenda with few ideas from the floor and little process, that is a sign. If your voice is the only voice across the table, take a hint. If the eyes around you are dull and discouraged and the only answers are single-word, three-lettered moans ("Yes"), pay heed. Pay heed, because if there's not already a steady stream of staff out the door, there soon will be. Look in the mirror and ask, "Am I the cause of this?"

I close this chapter with such remarks for a good reason. After supervising and coaching for a period of time, you are now ready to address the performance appraisal. All previous discussions with your employee are now precipitated into a crystallized dialogue that winds up on paper in a personnel file. Arrogance on your part will stifle this process.

MORSELS

The newest computer can merely compound, at speed, the oldest problem in relations between human beings, and in the end the communicator will be confronted with the old problem, of what to say and how to say it.

—Edward R. Murrow

7

Performance Appraisal: Where It All Comes Together

A Look at What You'll Learn:

- How to change a weapon into a useful alignment tool

- Why appraisal should be an ongoing process

- How to keep track of significant events

- How to enlarge and enrich the jobs of your employees

- Why self, peer, and other sources of input are so valuable

- How to conduct a performance appraisal session

- Why paper trails are so essential

- Where, when, and how to use reverse appraisal systems

A Tool, Not a Weapon

Few things strike more fear in the hearts of workers than performance appraisals. Symptoms abound: sweaty palms, nervous laughter, even out-of-body experiences. The poor aide withers before you, her confidence waning by the moment, as she awaits the guillotine that will slam down to erase her future. You look up from your papers, bite your lip, and sigh, "Hey, Jan! This is gonna be *great!*"

A performance appraisal does not have to be a harrowing experience. After all, the instrument is supposed to be a *tool*, not a *weapon*. The process itself celebrates the culmination of the most recent work period with a comprehensive review of not only the work performance, but the relationships surrounding the work, including the one between the supervisor and supervisee. It is a chance to take a look at everything related to the job at one time: the person, the peers, the team, the job, the facility, the training, the goals, even the organization. I prefer to think of it as an *up-raisal,* an educational experience, a chance to grow.

Despite their misgivings about the process, workers *do* want formal feedback. It validates their accomplishments and affords them new paths for future behavior and work. It helps to level the organizational chart by saying, "Hey, you are important to us! You count!" The appraisal adds credibility to your work as a supervisor and to the overall organization by serving as a landmark; time doesn't just march on, it has events anchored in writing, and this is one of them. The written document serves as the fiber linking work performance to personnel records, an assurance that a permanent record is on file for future reference.

You say, "That's fine if it's a *good* performance appraisal. What about the bad ones?" Good question. In my experience in this business, only about 1 in 20 appraisals is truly a "bad" one. This is partly due to the fact that truly poor employees rarely make it to the formal appraisal stage of the game; they drop out or are terminated before this juncture is reached. This is almost always true for the annual appraisal and occasionally for the 3-month appraisal, which used to be called the end of the probationary period. If an underperformer *is* around for an evaluation, it will most likely not be the gleeful experience I described above; *growthful* perhaps, but not gleeful.

On your side of the table, the performance appraisal is an excellent opportunity to bring all of your management skills to bear at once. It's like picking the fruit from the seed you planted in Chapter 5. You can now consolidate those hours of discussion and observation into one document and move on to the next stage of employee development. You get to test your personality-reading skills and see if you are even close in your original assessments. If you are facing the appraisal of a successful employee, you can validate that positive self-message you kept deep inside when the hire was completed (i.e., "This person is going to be a winner!").

If It Is a Surprise, It Is a Symptom

In training supervisors in this area of the work, I always make it a point to say, "If the employee is genuinely surprised at the tone of the performance appraisal (either positive *or* negative), you have not done your job well." There should be no big news at this juncture. If there is, you should take it as a symptom of failed communication; you have either not met regularly, avoided direct feedback, or both. Significant issues should *never* be stored by a supervisor for delivery on D day. Problems should be solved as they happen, and accolades should be bestowed on those who excel at the time of the excellence. One supportive instrument I like to use is the key incident journal, a copy of which is included in Appendix 2. If you jot down a few notes on occurrences during the year as they happen, you will have a ready reference come performance appraisal time. It makes no difference whether the key incident was good or bad—just pull out your journal and record the event.

Another Realignment Opportunity

As mentioned earlier, the performance appraisal joins hiring, meetings, and one-to-one supervision or coaching as an opportunity to realign expectations. In fact, it is the *best* of opportunities, because it is more focused and both retroactively and proactively positioned; you get the time to catch your breath and discuss what happened as you prepare to plan for what will be.

Very rarely do things stay the same in this business. By the time you perform an annual these days, the employee could have changed supervisors twice, across three work settings. The team may have changed its composition, and the work itself might be focused on a different population. I witnessed this at CMT one year, when the company added group homes to its list of clients. Therapists who had formerly done nothing but geriatric work in long-term care settings were suddenly treating severe cases of cerebral palsy, brain injuries, and developmental disabilities in private homes. When each employee's year ended, a matrix appraisal was performed by two supervisors (in most cases) to capture the entire year of work.

Because of the constant change in the industry, performance appraisals have had to take on new looks recently. The focus is increasingly on relationship development, the ability to adapt, attitude, and documentation, and less on actual clinical skills. This is a natural consequence, I feel, and not necessarily a good one. Although I endorse a strong focus on the interactive and attitudinal aspects, I fear that the clinical focus may be slipping away. Between managed care and multiple work sites, the industry is under pressure to maintain its clinical quality. Also, as mentioned, a thorough appraisal might require the work of two, even three, supervisors to be fair and accurate. It gets quite complicated when these supervisors disagree about the quality of the performance they are reviewing. Also, there is considerable concern about dilution because of cross-discipline supervision (PTs supervising OTs, SLPs supervising PTs, etc.). While I share this worry, I also realize that the marketplace will, for financial reasons, push this design on the industry even more in the future.

Rather than fighting change, you are better off to roll with it. Use it as a medium in your performance discussions. How has the job changed? How has the facility changed? How has the team changed? What changes does the employee see in herself or himself? Be careful not to let the *changes* become the complete focus, but don't ignore them either. Also, beware of the employee who uses *change* as an excuse for poor performance. Change is now the norm; sameness is the exception.

The setting of goals during the performance appraisal is just as important as the review of previous performance. I generally like to set six to eight goals with my employees, because that number offers variety without causing them to feel overwhelmed. You will notice that I used the term "*with* my employees," not "*for* my employees." Goal setting, under most circumstances, should be generated and agreed on mutually to maximize creativity and buy-in.

Job enlargement and *job enrichment* are two design concepts you might consider when setting goals to motivate future behavior. Job enlargement involves expanding the content of a job by increasing the number and variety of tasks performed. An example in our work might be the adding of patient screens to the job description of an aide, assuming that the work environment allows such activity at that level. Sure, it might be an additional task added to an otherwise full job, but it could also be an addition of considerable interest to the aide. Rearranging the assignment of caseloads to allow this aide to stay with patients she picked up through the screening process and making her responsible for the logistics of the treatment episode would be an example of job *enrichment*. This is similar to the enrichment that occurred in the automotive industry several years ago, when the switch was made from assembly *lines* to assembly *teams*. It was found that the quality of work life was much better when a worker was involved with a team assembling a complete door, for example, than with merely screwing in the same part, time after time. The satisfaction of standing back and looking at a whole job done well brings a more global feeling of satisfaction.

Job enrichment enables workers to perform not only more varied tasks, but tasks at a higher level—ones that give them greater responsibility for their work. We see enlargement and enrichment in clerical work all the time. What used to be "secretary" jobs are now advertised as "administrative assistants" in a move to enlarge and enrich jobs not only in title, but in function. Office managers realized that mere typing and answering the phone did not motivate people as much as performing administrative functions, such as handling projects, setting up educational events, and coordinating conference calls. As variety and responsibility were added, productivity increased.

Valuable Review Resources

In the old days, supervisors simply sat down, wrote up what they thought, and then handed the document to the employee, along with either a pay increase or a pink slip. We have come a long way since then. The modern approach—especially in our industry—is more collegial, more of a dialogue. Here are the review resources I find to be valuable and that I recommend you pursue:

The Performance Appraisal Instrument

The actual vehicle provided for you to assess performance can range from a blank sheet to a small book. I have employed many instruments within that range and find that there are a few merits, but several deficits, in the two extremes.

With the blank sheet, you can create your own standards, figure a way to measure against those standards, and then design a reward system to fit. This can be fun and fine if you (1) are quite creative, (2) have the time, (3) don't mind having to start from scratch every time, and (4) want to be all over the map with a different approach to each employee.

At the other pole is the 2-lb performance booklet. Many hospitals adopted this approach in the late 1980s when personnel consultants were convincing HR departments that every activity on a job description needed to appear on the performance appraisal instrument as a measurable activity. Rehabilitation teams all over the country spent months in this anal-retentive dissection of jobs, to the point of being ridiculous. While thoroughness is certainly attained, it has its price. I once saw a form for PTs that was 26 pages long *before* it had been filled out! It was exhausting just to look at it!

A performance appraisal model is included in Appendix 3. It is specifically designed for performance appraisal in rehabilitation in medical settings, so a stretch might be required to apply it in a school setting. If you work with a hospital, nursing home, or home-care company (particularly if it is part of a chain), you most likely have a generic instrument that applies to many different jobs. I urge you to attempt to modify that instrument toward a model that fits your work. Many nursing-based instruments are good and fairly close, but not with the exact focus you need for optimum results in the rehabilitation arena.

Self-Appraisal

A century ago, I would have been laughed off these pages for suggesting that employees be allowed to assess their own performance; now it is quite common. Self-appraisal has many positive payoffs. First, the employee's own opinion becomes part of the formal record, as opposed to the traditional approach, in which only the supervisor is allowed to comment. Second, the employee's comments might bring new information into the picture that the supervisor never knew about or understood. Finally, self-appraisal breeds responsibility and growth. By having to describe accomplishments and measure one's own performance, an employee gets another taste at a managementlike function.

I have managed in three companies for which self-appraisal scores actually contributed to the total score on which merit increases were rewarded. In a highly professional business like health care, I find this to be a mature approach. It represents a strong message from management about trust in the individual, and, by far, most employees act responsibly. Actually, as you might expect, most people *underrate* themselves in comparison to their peers and supervisors. When this occurs, I use it as the basis for a counseling session on improving self-esteem. When the opposite occurs—*overrated* self-measurement—another type of discussion emerges, one that focuses on self-perception, responsiveness to feedback, and (perhaps) humility. In either case, the self-appraisal leads to valuable and necessary lessons.

Peer Appraisal

As the externally imposed changes hit the industry, you will find yourself increasingly dependent on peer input during the evaluation of your employees' performances. The simple fact is this: You aren't always going to be there to observe performance. As the span of control grows to five or six supervisees, you will be forced to rely on formal input from others—therapists, assistants, and aides—to be able to formulate a well-rounded view of performance and attendant behaviors of the employee being evaluated.

Beyond this "extended lens," peer input strengthens the fabric of teams. If it becomes the norm for employees to formally participate in each others' performance appraisal, day-to-day communication tends to increase. An awareness that cooperation and coordination with a peer might affect your merit increase via input from that peer enhances positive behaviors. Also, encouraging peers to share what they wrote in a peer appraisal—a suggestion I always make—helps to establish the habit of providing face-to-face feedback during the rest of the work year.

I like to involve at least three peers in the appraisal process. When the time comes, I negotiate with my supervisee on the choices and attempt to assemble a good mix of people. I usually know who is close to whom and will suggest that all levels of staff be included; in this context, the word *peer* is not technically accurate, because we are not restricted to having employees of the same discipline or licensure serving as "peers."

One caution here: Look out for the "all or none" peer appraisal. This is the one with all of the highest or all of the lowest scores checked off, usually without comment. I *always* send these back to the perpetrator, because no one is *all* bad or *all* good. If a peer cannot justify such scores with thoughtful comments, I don't want her or his participation. I will ask the employee to choose another peer—one who pays some heed to the importance of this task.

Other Professionals

There are times when I go outside of the company to get additional feedback on an employee. This is normally when there are not enough company peers to meet the need, or a particular behavior problem with outside staff has been identified. For example, I once had an SLP whose interactions with her DON left something to be desired. I asked the DON to complete an abbreviated version of our peer instrument to get her input on paper, even though her scores on the criteria were not formally incuded in the total peer score. I find that when this occurs, outside people are very obliging and seem to appreciate having been asked to participate. And by the way, it is important to inform the employee of your intention to gather this information; otherwise, it gives the appearance of a witch hunt.

I recommend starting the peer and self-appraisal process 3 weeks before the scheduled performance appraisal meeting. If you hand out the forms at this time, allowing 2 weeks for return, you will have a whole week to consolidate all of the input into the final document.

Hard Copy

The following is a list of hard-copy resources that should be available to you before you write a comprehensive performance appraisal.

- **Job description(s).** Remember to retrace the trail for the period of the review. Has there been more than one job assignment this year? More than one job description?

- **Other key written agreements.** Sometimes, with contract staff, we forget to do an annual performance review. There is no reason not to use the same instrument you use for regular employees, but you might want a copy of the contract to peruse during the process.

- **Key incident journal.** As mentioned earlier, a log of the significant positive and negative events from the period of review is very helpful; see Appendix 2 for a sample.

- **Last year's/period's appraisal.** If this is not the first review, you should have the last one completed on hand to compare progress with goals. I also find it instructive to do a quick review of the previous document, just to see what issues were being discussed in the past.

- **Training log.** Some supervisors keep ongoing records of training received, a useful resource during reviews. You might check to see if rehabilitation administration or HR keeps such records.

- **New credential list.** If you or your company keeps track of credentials as they are added, it is nice to have that information available. Examples might be an MBA, a certification for hand therapy, or certification in athletic training, and so on. It is not only a good idea to make note of such accomplishments in the written appraisal, it might actually fit into the merit increase formula.

Amalgamation

If you are able to assemble all of the above resources, you are in a good position to write a thorough performance appraisal. We all have our own styles, and I do not want to impose mine on you. However, I think there is some logic in reviewing all of the sources of input before beginning your own written appraisal. This is particularly important if the employee being evaluated does not receive copies of the peer input and must rely on your *summarized* words. Similarly, if you do not read the *self*-appraisal before writing, you are basically ignoring all of that input, rendering it useless and a waste of the employee's time.

Besides the actual content of the written appraisals (self- and peer), I look for trends and themes. Is the feedback from the peers consistent? Is it drastically different than the self-appraisal? Am I seeing an attitude problem here or a lack of clinical skill?

Are the peers trying to tell me something without coming right out and saying it? Do I need to pull together a team meeting because of what I'm reading? Do I need to suggest to a peer that he or she confront the employee being evaluated because of the severity of what has been written?

I made a personal choice several years ago to write my appraisals as if I were speaking to the employee in person. Instead of writing, "Mary Smith has had an excellent year," I prefer, "You have had a great year, Mary." This helps the employee engage me and the feedback I have gathered in a more personal fashion. Speaking in a third-person tone tends to make employees feel less special; in my mind, they are *all* special.

To protect the confidentiality of the peers, I avoid describing specific incidences and generalize the trends—both positive and negative—into behavioral terms. I shy away from saying things like, "It has been noted that you frequently..." or "People who contributed say that you..." Instead, I try to weight the feedback as much as possible and be honest about its source. If I am making the observation, I own it, with, "It is my observation that..." or "In my opinion..." With peers, I often write, "The peer input was consistent in saying that you..." or, "One of your peers noted that you..." I will also refer to the self-appraisal at times with comments like, "I noticed that you join your peers and me in observing that you..." or, conversely, "The fact that your own opinion on this was in direct contrast to that of your peers tells me that..."

An enormous amount of cortical activity occurs when you are amalgamating seven or eight sources of information into one document (i.e., hard copy from the past, peer and self-input, your own observations). You must consider both the past and the future, the team and extended team(s), your own performance as the supervisor and coach, the frailty or strength of the employee, and the valence of the reward or reprimand. For this reason, I suggest a quiet writing location, where interruptions will be at a minimum. Many supervisors do their appraisals at home, and I think that is an excellent idea— unless you have two hungry kids, a barking dog, a city utilities truck idling on the street in front of the house, and two ringing phones, as I do this very minute.

Delivery

D day has arrived. You have been respectful to your employee by completing everything 1 week before the due date; thus HR will get everything in time for the appropriate paperwork to be completed. To ensure a thorough reading of the written document, you have given the written performance appraisal to the employee yesterday afternoon or perhaps this morning. You come out from behind your desk (or mat, or charting table) and sit face-to-face, with no barriers between you. If you notice a growing ring of wetness just below the armpits, you put the employee at ease by saying, "Relax, this is going to be fun. It was good year," or "You look a little uptight. We have some challenges this time, but nothing we can't work out."

Taking the time to calm your employee is worthwhile. Even the strongest of our employees knows that she or he is on the downside of the power differential, and the performance appraisal *feels* like one gigantic button in the hand of a super-parent. Anything you can do to bring relaxation and focus is helpful. I have had people so freaked out that they barely remembered the content on the day after the meeting.

Complete the process by summarizing the highlights, reviewing the goals, and congratulating good performers for a job well done. Be sure that they sign the original and their own copy and date both documents.

About Paper Trails . . .

The emphasis on copies, signatures, and dates on important documents like performance appraisals relates to paper trails. If you are a new grad and have just finished your paper *chase,* you probably don't even want to hear about paper of any kind. That is understandable, but paper of the trail type can save your butt—and the butt of your company. Paper trails are those critical documents that either keep you out of court or save you when you get there. Issues of conflict such as discrimination (age, gender, race, lifestyle), wrongful discharge, and harassment are often debated in court not on what was said, but what was *written.* Hiring letters, memos to file, letters of warning, and final notices of corrective action are typical examples of important paper. Therefore, you must be careful to be honest, accurate, consistent, and of good intentions in your personnel-related documentation. For example, getting angry on paper is not as effective as getting precise, in behavioral terms, about what needs to change. Getting even is worse. We don't always know if what we are writing will end up in court, so it is a good idea to assume that *everything* will end up there. When creating a piece of writing that will become a footprint on the paper trail, be sure that you are calm and collected. If you are concerned about its content and style, have an HR representative (or your CEO or other administrator) review the document before giving it to the employee.

I want to close by making a connection between performance appraisals and paper trails that might get you a nice kiss on the forehead from your local HR representative. I have a phrase—"motivational appraisal"—to describe the scenario in which a supervisor gives an inflated evaluation to a substandard employee in the hope that good scores will increase motivation. I normally see this occur not with the really poor employee, but with the marginal ones, the ones who just don't quite measure up.

Motivational appraisals are a no-no for two big reasons. First, they are not honest, and they merely validate unacceptable behavior or performance. Second, they litter the paper trail. Nothing is more infuriating to an HR rep than to have a therapist march in and demand the firing of an aide, only to find out that a good (motivational) performance appraisal was just completed on that aide 3 months earlier. Yet we see this happen all the time. By trying to massage a weak employee into conformity with unrealistically high scores, all you do is contaminate the process. It is much, much more effective to be straight at the time, to identify the deficiencies, and to set goals. If corrective action is needed to get her or his attention, use it. Don't do sweet talk on paper.

MORSELS

Perhaps the most innovative and daring instrument I have ever worked with is the reverse performance appraisal. Going beyond self- and peer input, this approach actually allows supervisees to formally evaluate their jobs, their supervisors, and the company. The implementation of reverse performance appraisal requires a work system of openness and honesty, where management is eager to learn and grow. Here are the steps involved:

1. The employee feedback form contains a section for written evaluation of the job, the immediate supervisor, and the company at large (or department, if that is more pertinent). Questions are fairly broad, allowing the evaluator the freedom to state what he or she thinks and feels.

2. The instrument is applied during the performance appraisal of each supervisee. By taking this approach, feedback is generated regularly throughout the year, rather than just once, when the supervisor is being evaluated by his or her superior.

3. The written portion of the employee feedback form is completed before the performance appraisal session.

4. During the performance appraisal session, the supervisor proceeds as she or he normally would, evaluating the work of the supervisee for the previous period, while leaving time for the feedback session.

5. During the feedback session, the supervisee goes over the written form and turns it in to the supervisor.

6. The feedback form is then sent to the next highest level of supervision for review (in our industry, this would be the program manager, regional manager, etc.). That manager then decides if a meeting with the supervisor is in order due to the content of the feedback form.

7. The form then moves up the line to the highest level of leadership so that feedback on the company itself can be shared.

8. The feedback form is never copied or filed. Once it reaches the top, it is returned to the originating employee, with signatures proving that all appropriate levels of the organization became involved in this process.

The reverse performance appraisal system seems cumbersome and threatening to many people. While this system does require additional time and effort, I submit that the payoff is unparalleled in terms of strengthening the vertical communication of any company that dares to install it.

8

Vocational Divorce:
When It Doesn't Work Out

A Look at What You'll Learn:

- The terminology of human resources
- How to use corrective action when performance issues arise
- Types of separation from work and when to consider them
- How to use resignation as an alternative to termination
- How to conduct an employee termination session
- Paper trails, exit interviews, and other helpful tools

In spite of all that we do, there are times when it just doesn't work out with an employee: The fit was never good, the employee changed, the job changed, the organization changed, or perhaps the supervision was poor. I have seen work conflict recently because the *industry* changed. We will continue to see more problems related to such changes for the reasons already cited. If these problems lead to divorce, we need to be prepared to make that divorce as amicable as possible.

Corrective Action

In these days of political correctness, *corrective action* has replaced the more negative terminology of yesteryear. Thirty years ago, people were put on probation, and if their performance didn't improve fairly soon, they were fired without much in the way of intervening steps. Today, thankfully, there are many processes designed to protect employees from unfair labor practices. If an employee's continued employment is in jeopardy, we are obliged to counsel and supply formal warning if significant personnel action is pending. Collectively, these activities constitute corrective action.

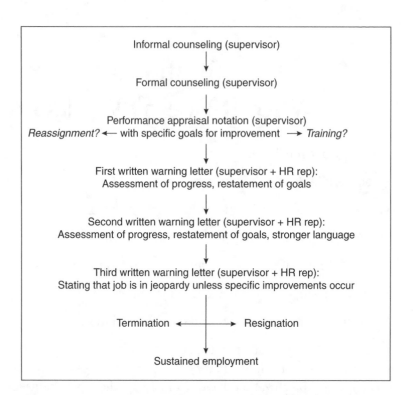

FIGURE 8-1. Typical steps in corrective action. The exact sequence and number of events that occur during corrective action are dependent on the policies of the company. The purpose of such steps is to allow fair and adequate warning to the employee, while offering specific information on remediation of the problem(s). As shown, the language of each step becomes more severe as possible termination looms. Because a paper trail is laid down during this process, supervisors are advised to consult with HR (or personnel) office experts once the formal counseling stage is reached.

Figure 8-1 provides a sequence of corrective action steps that might appear in the procedure manual of the HR department in a large organization. The list varies from company to company, even from state to state, because of differences in local personnel law. However, be aware that the protections afforded employees by the Equal Employment Opportunities Commission (EEOC) require that employers proceed cautiously in dealing with personnel issues to assure nondiscriminatory treatment. If you work for a small company that lacks such protocols, be sure to consult an attorney before taking formal remedial action.

Lawyer or no lawyer, there are several commonsense things you need to know about corrective action. First, it is *highly* confidential in nature, and breaches on your part are not only ungainly, they are illegal. You are dealing with core issues related to a human being's livelihood, promotion, or demotion, and there is little sympathy for a loose tongue. Remedial activities in the personnel arena are touchy, technical, and potentially litigious in nature. For these reasons, it is a good idea to invite a witness to most meetings related to formal corrective action for the protection of both parties.

Counseling, memos, warning letters, performance appraisal notations, and the like are intended to inform the employee of existing problems while providing a plan of action to correct those problems. Employees deserve a fair and reasonable chance at improving performance or changing attitudes, with assistance from training or reassignment if necessary. Suspension with or without pay is an option that is invoked at times, usually when an illegal or life-threatening action has occurred.

Then comes the paper trail. You don't like to think of yourself as a schemer—out to get some poor helpless soul who isn't making it— but you are responsible, in fact, for documenting each and every step of corrective action. It just goes with the territory. In large organizations, HR will assist you with this, but in small ones you might be on your own. Just be sure to record accurate notes, dates, agreements, and all involved parties; get signatures when you can; and provide copies to the employee. If corrective action leads to termination, you will be glad you have this documentation to support the action you have taken, should there be litigation.

Types of Separation

To assist you with the vernacular, here is a short list of current terms used by HR folks to describe the various types of vocational divorce, along with a few paper trail pointers.

- **Termination for cause.** A forced separation from employment because of performance, illegal/unethical acts, violations of policies and procedures, and so forth. Termination requires the tightest paper trail in anticipation of possible litigation. In contemporary personnel management practice—except in cases in which an illegal, unethical, or life-threatening activity has occurred—the standard paper trail is fairly long. It includes a combination of performance appraisal documentation (at least one document), followed by letters of warning—the number of which depends on company policy and the severity of the situation. The final letter includes "final warning" terminology, along with specifics as to what behavior or performance needs to improve and by when. Termination for cause should always be accompanied by a carefully crafted letter from an HR representative or an attorney.

- **Resignation.** A voluntary separation initiated by the employee. Not normally a high-risk action, unless the employee can prove duress or harassment. It is wise to document any meetings related to the resignation and to obtain a resignation letter for the files.

- **Reduction in force.** This is the modern term for a layoff of personnel, either temporarily or permanently. Applicable to one position or more, it will become a more frequent occurrence in an industry that has had little need for cutbacks in the past 20 years. Again, precise terminology on notices and letters to the employee(s) is critical.

- **Elimination of position.** This is a sister to reduction in force, with a slight twist. In this case, the position itself is also removed. The same rules regarding accuracy of notification apply.

- **Suspension.** As mentioned earlier, suspension is an action available to supervisors in certain situations. Suspensions are used either punitively or as a means of removing the employee from the work environment during an investigation. Some suspensions become either terminations for cause or resignations, whereas others are resolved with no further action. Examples of behavior leading to suspension include alleged theft, intoxication on the job, violence, serious breach of procedures, endangerment of a patient or staff member, and chronic absenteeism or tardiness. Careful documentation is required.

- **Retirement.** This one's just thrown in here to be complete. Remember to celebrate!

Resignation as an Option

I would venture to say that I have had to actually *terminate* (fire) only six or seven employees in my career as a manager. Each of these involved extreme circumstances, in which I felt that the employee had given me (or the company) no chance to maneuver and salvage the situation. Once, in the mid-1970s, a counselor scheduled a community dance under the name of my company, without my knowledge, and allowed kids to smoke marijuana on the premises. This counselor was working in a substance abuse prevention program. Another involved an Adult Protective Services social worker who made sexual advances toward the widow of his former client, on the grave of the deceased, on company time (not too weird!). Probably the worst one was an SLP I had to excommunicate on the phone. This was a woman who had a long-standing history of difficulty with her supervisors; her refusal to attend an afternoon meeting with me and her then-supervisor led to her demise via AT&T. For your information, this was in a hospital setting, and it followed four phone calls and three trips by me to HR. I didn't give up on her easily.

There are times when things don't have to go that way. I don't relish cutting people loose, and I always feel a sense of personal failure when this happens. What more could I have done? Did I really understand all of the angles? When I found out that the SLP I fired on the phone was a single mom, I felt absolutely terrible. But then I realized that I had done everything I could to get her to understand the severity of the situation. The final two calls included clear warnings about an imminent termination if she failed to show up for the meeting. This followed several warning letters and other meetings with her supervisor in which no discernible progress was made.

Sometimes resignation is an option to termination—I have probably convinced two dozen people to resign during my career. There are simply times when *fit* is the issue, not *attitude*. An employee might have excellent people skills, but the deficits in clinical skills cannot be tolerated. After a long process of attempting remediation, termination or resignation is the only option.

I had this very situation several years ago with an assistant who had tested for his certificate in another state and then practiced across the border. His previous jobs as a rehab tech had afforded him considerable hands-on experience, but the fundamental knowledge of physiology and anatomy was simply not there. After 6 months of attempting to gear him up through evening classes failed, I was forced to negotiate his resignation. This was a person I truly liked, and it was very painful. On the other hand, it was my job to protect the patients, and I felt that they were at risk in the hands of an untrained assistant. We remain friends.

Perhaps many managers would have simply fired the assistant in the example I just gave. I suppose it is quicker, maybe even easier, for some people. But from my experience, very little learning goes on during terminations. People leave feeling abused, misunderstood, and with little to go on when they approach a new job. As I did with the assistant, I try to offer a lens through which the situation might be viewed differently. The work experience wasn't a failure, and the separation wasn't a personal rejection. Several times I have managed to get departing employees to realize that many risks surrounded their continued employment with my company: medical and legal risks with regard to the patient or client, perhaps personal exposure. With rare exception, I have found these attempts to educate to be met with respect and appreciation. I'm not saying that they were fun (on either side of the table), but they were *fair*.

A couple of words of caution. Before you run out and convince someone to resign, be sure that your paper trail is in order, should he or she refuse your advice. Not everyone is receptive to such an option, and some people will resent you for even suggesting resignation. You don't want to *force* a resignation. Also, be sure to check with HR before taking this approach; some companies have specific policies regarding terminations and resignations, and you want to be aligned with those policies. Also, there are unemployment insurance implications.

The Termination Session

Nothing keeps me awake at night more than knowing I must terminate someone the next day. Fortunately, as I said, it has been a rare occurrence, and I would like to keep it that way. I would much prefer to put my energy into effective hiring and supervision.

There are a few standard procedures to consider when facing a termination session. First, as mentioned, you should invite a witness and be sure that all of your paperwork is in order. All salary and benefit-related moneys should be paid at the time, including outstanding reimbursements for mileage, meals, or supplies. If there is any thought of a potential for violence, you might post an additional person outside the door (security, if in a hospital or school).

Keep the termination session short and sweet. Don't be mean or vindictive, just even tempered and clear. If Consolidated Omnibus Budget Reconciliation Act (COBRA) rights (i.e., rights to continued medical and dental benefits) and other HR-related issues need to be explained, refer the employee to the appropriate person and show him or her to the door.

While some termination sessions are amicable, most are not. It is best to say as little as possible, because the more you say, the more you are likely to either spark anger or get you and your company into some kind of legal problem. Let the writing do most of the talking and try to keep your mouth shut.

Turnover Rates

Most health care entities experience annual turnover rates in the 15–25% range. Figures in the upper register can be indicative of organizational problems, but not always. Ours is an industry that couples a relatively young work force with great opportunity to travel and see the country; therefore, turnover rates are affected by voluntary resignation. The *reasons* for those resignations can be extracted from exit interviews. Are people leaving a bad situation or merely choosing to take advantage of the chance to travel while they are young and free? It pays to know.

Divorce Done Well

Separation from employment can be like a divorce: done good, done bad, or done ugly. The process is often sober, and the results can be unsatisfying. On the other hand, good management is an active process of moving people into and out of jobs, and something you must get used to. If you apply the principles and stay true to your heart and your company, you will be fine. I occasionally run into people whose departures I have hastened, through legislated resignation, and rarely find one who isn't better off for having moved along.

MORSELS

Separation from employment is ripe with barbs. Between equal opportunity employers, the Americans with Disabilities Act (ADA), union protections, and state merit laws that support public employees, you have a narrow margin for error in dealing with separation—particularly when forced termination of employment is involved. Lawyers may be expensive, but a quick consult before you take separation action with an employee is much less costly than the court action that might follow.

III   It's About Time!

In the CMT survey, time management was chosen as one of the top three challenges facing contemporary therapists. That probably comes as no surprise to you. Your day is a rushed, rapid-fire blur of meetings, evaluations, treatments, supervisory sessions, attempts to get orders, trips across town, flurries of cryptic documentation, and unanswered phone calls—a flight interrupted only by the crises that make it all worse. Catch-up happens in the middle of the night, when you fly from your bed crying, "Oh my God! Did I take that hot pack off Mrs. Muggilicutty?"

Don't feel persecuted. We all suffer with the time crunch. As a matter of fact, there are few subjects more difficult to discuss than the management of one's time. This is because personal time management is a highly individualized, highly situational phenomenon. No simple answer, no single formula exists for those who suffer with problems related to time; the solutions lie in your personality and lifestyle, and, not surprisingly, they are difficult to find because you lack the time to search for them! This is the cycle of time deprivation that keeps most of us rambling along, doing things the same old way, feeling one step behind.

Time management is a philosophy, not a technique. In this book, that philosophy is presented as *self*-management, because time itself is only a structure within which we schedule our lives. We don't really manage time, we manage ourselves, *within time*, by prioritizing our activities.

In this part, we will first take another look at you and how you manage yourself (Chapter 9) and then deal with the external variables that you can affect in the effort to enhance the efficiency of your team (Chapter 10).

9

Proper Focus

A Look at What You'll Learn:

- Why time management is really self-management
- How your own personal and professional habits affect efficiency
- A better way of thinking about crises and priorities
- A model for choosing appropriate activities to save time

Because gourmet cooking is one of my hobbies, I thought I would begin this chapter with a recipe. Let's call it "Recipe for a Bad Day."

Ingredients:

15 gallons of gasoline (in the car, on the way to a 7:00 AM meeting with a physician, because you forgot to fill the tank last night; makes you 10 minutes late)

12 oz coffee (to wake up from lack of sleep caused by worrying about a quality assessment [QA] report due at the end of the week)

Dash across town (to pick up a soft chart that couldn't be found on the third floor of the other hospital yesterday)

Pinch of customer service (to soothe a patient angry about being charged full fare for a treatment performed by an assistant)

1 tbs of tears (collected from a technician feeling abused by a fellow therapist)

Slice of life (listening to a long-winded tirade from a foreign-trained therapist who is in danger of being deported because she failed to renew her visa)

1 ton of crushed feelings (from a 6-year-old daughter whose first-grade play somehow failed to make the calendar)

Simmering crisis in rehabilitation meeting (because nurses and therapists are fighting about access to patients in the morning hours)

Minced words with program manager (for failing to mention that the QA report was also supposed to be presented orally to the medical director in an unannounced meeting on Friday morning)

Two crabs (a pair of patients who don't want to follow home instruction packets)

A parsley-completed meeting with a valued sage named Rosemary (cut short for lack of thyme)

One half-baked proposal (for a new workers' compensation program; returned by administration with some less-than-complimentary comments attached)

2 lb of frustration (because the hot pack machine went down at noon and the backup was loaned to outpatient a week ago)

Skimmed review of progress notes (because there isn't time for a thorough reading)

Grated nerves (because the *International Classification of Diseases–9 Code Book* can't be found and billing wants to wrap up the month)

Sour grapes (from a peer who didn't get promoted to senior staff status)

Shredded emotions (from a hastily assembled team meeting at the end of the day called to announce the loss of a veteran PTA)

Cooking instruction: Blend for 9 hours in a job that is half therapist, half supervisor.

Yield: One toasted professional (a Crispy Critter)

When this kind of day is *your* day, there is no joy of cooking. You go home resentful and angry, feeling like the world beat up on you the minute you left home. Then you start blaming time for your troubles.

Time management isn't really about time at all, it's about you and the choices you make. Time is nothing more than a box into which we cram events. If you estimate the capacity of the box well, size the events accurately, and then stack your activities in the proper order, you're fine. If, on the other hand, you underestimate the size of the box, try to put too much stuff in it or get the stuff out of order, you have a mess. You're late. Things don't get done. You look disorganized. People lose confidence. The box may change because of the size and shape of your job, but it is still just a vessel, a measure called *time*; it can hold many small events or a few big ones, wrong activities or right ones. In the end, however, it is the stuffer who makes the choices, not the box.

The questions are many: Are you a good time box stuffer? Do you make good choices? Do you prioritize well? Do you plan? Do you have control over what goes in your time box? If not, what percentage *do* you control?

For the past decade, I have heard therapists lament the lack of control they feel over time and, therefore, over their work lives. "It ain't the way it used to be!" they cry. If managed care isn't the culprit, it's the facility, the hospital, or the school system. Then there is the endless paperwork, not to mention the long list of languorous meetings. In speaking of time, I say it is time to stop externalizing the problem and look inward, where time management begins: with you.

I suspect that most of us developed our self-management habits as students. After all, we spent about 18 years in the student lifestyle that gelled when we entered junior high: daytime class work and nighttime homework, midnight cramming, and praying for multiple-choice tests. A carry-through to professional work habits seems almost inevitable. In fact, thinking about *study* habits as children (an exercise occasioned by our parents) might be the closest any of us ever got to evaluating the *work* habits we sustain as adults.

In spite of the path *you* took to get here, it is important to understand where you are in your own evolutionary process relative to time management. In Appendix 4 I have included a self-survey titled "Time Will Tell" to help you in the assessment of your status as a time manager. Take it now. Circle the appropriate responses, and total the score at the bottom. If your total score is 25 or above, you are probably quite good at managing your own time. If your total is 15 or below, read this section carefully. If the range is somewhere between 16 and 24, note those categories where you scored a "1" and pay particular attention to them during the ensuing discussions.

Evolving Toward Self-Management

To move from a *time* management mentality to one of *self*-management, you must evaluate two major areas of your work life:

1. How you organize yourself to accomplish activities, and

2. How you prioritize those activities.

There seems to be an evolutionary process at work in becoming self-managed. Figure 9-1 reflects the stages through which most of us evolve in the attempt to become more organized. Beginning at the upper left and moving clockwise, we see a progression of five stages, from the most basic approaches (mechanical) to the most sophisticated (proactive). The stages tend to be additive, such that a person at stage V is using some of the techniques from the earlier stages, even if all of them are not particularly effective. Few of us attain perfect efficiency. I am certain that you will see some of yourself in each stage, as I do.

Stage I. Early Mechanical: Stickies, Scraps, and Notes to Yourself

Otherwise known as *treasures of the pocket*, these are the ever-familiar reminders that we have all used in the faint hope that we might be able to translate our garble to action at some later date. My personal favorites are the incomplete notes, those little gems-in-progress that were interrupted by an unexpected distraction. Perhaps you have plucked a crumpled scrap from your own pocket or purse with scribbling that said something like *don't forget to remind the team about*

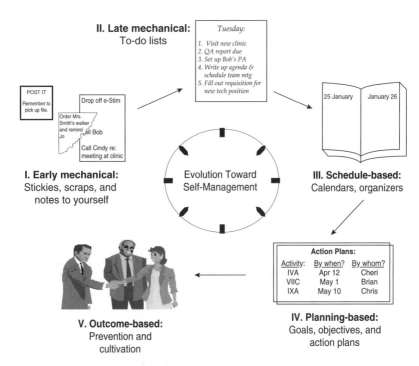

FIGURE 9-1. In the evolution toward self-management, one moves from physical reminders to planning, thinking, and proactive relationship-building activities. While most workers use some version of all five stages in their daily lives, managers must learn to increase their impact and efficiency by concentrating on the more advanced methods.

the meeting on. . . . Or how about that stickie pulled from the scheduling board that says *Important! Call Tim at 555-67. . . .*

Relying on such cryptic short stuff is not a recommended method for managing yourself. Virtually everyone (including me) resorts to this primitive approach at one time or another, but it has serious pitfalls. The information is scattered, subject to loss or destruction, and often illegible. It makes you look disorganized (because you are) and can cause you to lose the respect of your colleagues—particularly if mistakes and missed appointments result from your sloppy trail of tattered interpretations. If you are relying on this kind of paper trail to remain organized, you will have great difficulty being an effective therapist-supervisor.

Stage II. Late Mechanical: To-Do Lists

Ah, the infamous list of things to do! More advanced than scrappy notes and probably the most widely used tactic for staying organized, this approach can be helpful at times. However, to-do lists still constitute a rather basic form of time management, because they only serve to remind you of *what* we need to do, not *why* you need to do it. Also, if you lack a centralized method of self-organization, you are likely to lose the to-do list. It is wise, therefore, to identify a special location for *all* to-do lists that you create. Because you almost always share office, counter, charting, or home space with several other people, it is wise to choose a private location for which you can guarantee yourself security. Here are a few ideas.

- **Locations to avoid:** Communal surfaces (countertops, desks, file cabinet tops, etc.), desk drawers, scheduling boards, in/out baskets, walls, floor of the car, kitchen table at home, back of the toilet, and so on.

- **Locations to favor:** Isolated pocket of a purse, calendar or day-timer/organizer (written in or stapled in), well-labeled file in file cabinet, personal mail box or locker, personal well-labeled clipboard, and so on.

If they can be easily used, updated, checked off, and then destroyed, to-do lists are not by nature unacceptable. If, however, they become a pile of partially reviewed plans that are lost half of the time, to-do lists are counterproductive, because you spend more time looking for them (or questioning if they are completed) than you do using them.

Stage III. Schedule-Based: Calendars and Organizers

Although still fairly mechanical, the use of date books and sophisticated organizers is a significant step forward. With their clever ticklers and resource sections, these modern marvels of paper timekeeping can become the central nerve center of your work life. The combination of calendar, notepad, and resource sections afford us one-stop shopping in a portable information center. Depending on the model, you can plan out your week, month, or year and cross-reference your planning. The computerized versions include database functions that provide for instant merging and sorting if easy access to a computer is possible at work. Either type can be purchased at office superstores at a cost ranging from $40 to $100.

If you keep your own treatment schedule, the loss of a calendar or organizer can be devastating. Therefore, it is wise to take two simple precautions:

1. Enter your name, address, and phone number in the front section of the book in permanent ink. Offer a reward for the return if you really value the contents.

2. Use the stage II list for storing your book; don't leave it lying around. The high-end organizers are often leather bound, and replacement contents can be purchased rather cheaply, so they become attractive to the less than honest.

The first three stages are useful and prevalent, particularly for jobs that lack leadership responsibilities, because they tend to focus on *things* and *time*. For a manager, they constitute only the first few rungs on the ladder to self-management.

Stage IV. Planning-Based: Goals, Objectives, and Action Plans

When we begin to budget time for thoughtful planning, we usually see a significant increase in organization and efficiency. If those plans are translated into written goals, objectives, and time-based action plans, our role assignments and timelines are purposeful, and clarity begins to emerge. While it is important for all workers to find some time to think and plan, it is an *essential* requirement of those who supervise the work of others. With proper planning, we become more *proactive* in our approach and *initiate* activity rather than merely react to it. Poor planning (or *no* planning) always catches up with us, because mistakes are obvious and expensive (either financially, emotionally, or politically). Here are a few tips you might find helpful in trying to become a better planner:

- Don't get crazy about it. If you can identify a goal you want to attain, write it out clearly, and identify a *few* actions that will lead to the accomplishment of the goal (maybe three or four activities, not 15).

- Don't spend hours and hours on personal planning. Most of our plans are never carried out, because things change too quickly. If you can budget 15 minutes a week to plan, you will be far ahead of your peers.

- Write your plans down, don't keep them in your head. You can use your to-do list, the notepad section of your calendar or organizer, or a computer for this purpose. Just as the writing of this book causes me to clarify my thinking, writing out plans will help you to clarify yours.

Stage V. Outcome-Based: Prevention and Cultivation
The highest form of self-management is attained when we begin to adopt a strong outcome orientation to our work. This is accomplished by actually budgeting time to *think*. This is a difficult leap for most therapists because of the hands-on nature of the work; you literally work with your hands in providing patient care, so thinking time can feel like idle time. The fact is, however, that moving up the chain from supervision to management to administration means being paid more to think. The active anticipation of problems (prevention) and the purposeful development of key relationships (cultivation) require thinking that will promote harmony and reduce crises. As we will see in a moment, they also mean prioritizing your activities in new ways and attacking external variables that enhance efficiency for you and those you supervise.

With the exception of stage I, a combination of the remaining stages usually results in an organized work style, if you are organizing the right activities.

Doing What's Right: Urgency and Importance

Doing what's right is hindered by trying to do too much too fast. As a matter of fact, there are a number of negative consequences that emanate from rushing:

- Rushing causes us to make mistakes. In health care, those mistakes can be fatal.

- Rushing causes us to become short-tempered and irritable. Little mistakes become big ones, distractions become interruptions, and soon our day has deteriorated.

- Rushing causes us to become myopic and shortsighted; without having time to think, we do what is in front of us at the time and becomes more crisis oriented.

- Rushing makes us unapproachable and therefore inaccessible; an inaccessible supervisor is an ineffective supervisor.

- Rushing becomes a habit; once you have the habit, you feel that you are not doing anything useful if you are not rushing.

In his best-selling book, *The Seven Habits of Highly Effective People,* Stephen R. Covey* offers a time-management matrix (Figure 9-2) from which to study the relationships between urgency, importance, and time management.

The two principal factors, *urgency* and *importance,* define how we choose our activities. Urgent things act on us, whether or not they are important, if we allow them to. Important things have more to do with our personal values or company goals, and if they are not urgent, they require more proactivity to produce desired results.

If your personal style is to feel a sense of urgency about what is *important,* your activity falls mostly into quadrant I.* For some positions—like an ambulance driver or perhaps a NASA crisis manager—this might be the proper posture in the short-term sense. Over time,

---

*From The Seven Habits of Highly Effective People. Copyright 1989 Stephen R. Covey. Reprinted with permission. All rights reserved.

	URGENT	NOT URGENT
IMPORTANT	**I.** **Activities:** Crises Pressing problems Deadline-driven projects	**II.** **Activities:** Prevention, production-capability activities; relationship building; recognizing new opportunities; planning recreation
NOT IMPORTANT	**III.** **Activities:** Interruptions, some calls, some mail, some reports, some meetings; proximate, pressing matters; popular activities	**IV.** **Activities:** Trivia, busy work, some mail; some phone calls; time wasters; pleasant activities

FIGURE 9-2. The time-management matrix. Stephen R. Covey's model allows us to classify our daily activities according to their importance and urgency. Whether at work or at play, we make conscious and unconscious choices about what we do within this framework. Such choices are a reflection of both our habits and our values. (From The Seven Habits of Highly Effective People. Copyright 1989 Stephen R. Covey. Reprinted with permission. All rights reserved.)

however, quadrant I* people experience stress and burnout, leaving little time, energy, or interest for quadrant II or III* activities, which are urgent but unimportant or not urgent and important, respectively.

Health care has its fair share of quadrant I*–dominant types. These are the crisis-oriented folks who run hither and yon, putting out fires with an audible sense of purpose. Hyper-helpers can fall into this category, because valid crises bring an immediate sense of purpose, and the importance of the rescue validates them. Because

---

*From The Seven Habits of Highly Effective People. Copyright 1989 Stephen R. Covey. Reprinted with permission. All rights reserved.

they are so exhausted, they find relief in escaping to quadrant IV*
activities (not urgent, not important), which are of little or no
impact on the work to be accomplished.

The second of the crisis-oriented types are those who make quadrant
III* choices. These people always seem to be in a dither, but you never
really know quite why. The urgency they bring seems to have no foundation, because productive results rarely show. There is no time to pull back
and consider planning or strategizing, because everything feels like an
emergency to them. If one comes from a dysfunctional family background, it is easy to get caught in this time-management trap. Not used
to thinking long range, quadrant III* types want or need to be helpful,
but have difficulty prioritizing what is important. They feel unappreciated, because they work hard, but the crises never seem to end. A manager who role-models with this choice structure can be devastating.

Quadrant IV* activities are chosen by people that Covey
describes as "basically leading irresponsible lives." Not much analysis
is needed here, because these folks do not usually last long in health
care (or anywhere else, for that matter).

If you have not guessed it by now, quadrant II* is the heart of effective self-management. People who operate in this quadrant perform
activities that are important but not necessarily urgent because they *can*.
The reason they can is simple: *Quadrant II* people exert influence on the
work environment in a way that reduces or eliminates the urgency of their
activities.* Efficient people avoid quadrants* III and IV for obvious reasons and try to keep quadrant I activities to a minimum. This is done by
building strong work relationships, anticipating problems through preventive activities, and doing what it takes to enhance productivity.
Quadrant II* people stay organized by using stage II–V self-organization
techniques and avoid the traps of stage I (tattered notes and stickies).
Thus the desirable time management matrix looks like Figure 9-3, with
quadrant II* as the preferred choice for the efficient self-manager.

---

*From The Seven Habits of Highly Effective People. Copyright 1989
Stephen R. Covey. Reprinted with permission. All rights reserved.

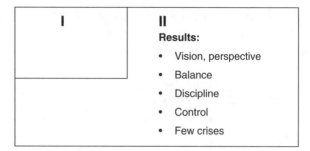

FIGURE 9-3. By choosing quadrant II activities on a regular basis, supervisors avoid the traps of crisis orientation and insignificant activity—two habits that rob them of effectiveness. The results shown here help bring harmony and success to the already harried lifestyle of the therapist-supervisor. (From The Seven Habits of Highly Effective People. Copyright 1989 Stephen R. Covey. Reprinted with permission. All rights reserved.)

To help explain the wisdom of self-management, I like to compare it with organic gardening. The basic theory behind organic gardening is that healthy soil grows stronger, more resistant plants, which in turn produce better crops. Healthy soil is gained by cultivation, recycling, mulching, and the deployment of compatible plants and animals in the surrounding garden. Much of this activity occurs before a seed is ever sown in anticipation of the benefits to the seedlings and mature plants. For the past 30 years I have prepared for planting by rototilling composted leaves and grass clippings into the ground before adding night crawlers and other worms to help ventilate the soil and distribute nutrients. I also add other animals and plants known to either feed on or deter unwanted pests: ladybugs, praying mantises, bacteria, umbels, and marigolds. This is followed by mulching with dead leaves and grass clippings to help warm the soil, hold in moisture, keep the weeds away, and maintain an on-ground composting process. Such cultivation and nurturing affords me a rich, loose loam into which plants can send long, strong, deep roots. At maturity, the stems are tougher, the vegetation is more lush, and the overall plant has a greater resistance to drought and disease—all because I took preventive measures and built a "relationship" with this plant.

The parallels with efficient self-management choices are fairly obvious. The cultivation of key relationships helps to prevent the development of crises, a chronic disease of time consumption. Proactive efforts to educate a broad range of staff as to how things are really done brings the organisms at work into a closer, more symbiotic relationship, and the team machine runs more smoothly. Planning is the mulching of the workplace to assure a continuous supply of needed resources, free of weedlike distractions.

Urgency Addiction

Those who fail to plan or prevent problems often suffer from "urgency addiction." Urgency addiction is a very difficult habit to change. Many people in health care are plagued with it, and a challenge to their priorities is perceived as an attack on their very souls. I have found this to be particularly true for some of those who work at the two ends of the age spectrum: pediatrics and geriatrics. To question knee-jerk attention to the plight of the very young or the very old—especially in crises—is like assailing motherhood and apple pie. For this reason, it is stressful for a supervising therapist to lean on an assistant or tech (or peer, for that matter) who races to the rescue every time a patients burps. And, of course, you might not even notice this tendency if you suffer from urgency addiction yourself.

The next time you find yourself putting out a fire, try to evaluate your motives. Are you intervening because you must or because it feels good? Is this something someone else could do for you? Did this crisis arise because of preventive measures you failed to take? Can you make a step toward an efficient, self-managed work lifestyle, or will you forever be dragging hose behind a siren?

MORSELS

When the "Just Say No" campaign hit the airways in the early 1980s, I just shook my head; I knew that preventing substance abuse was much more complicated than reciting a simple-minded slogan, and that few kids would turn down a joint because the president's wife had taught them a two-letter word. When I apply the idea to time management, however, I find that it has some merit. Many of us are simply too quick to help with things that could be done by others, and by rarely saying no, we fail to test the urgency of the events to which we respond so readily. True emergencies are rare. Try counting them on your fingers for 1 week and see if you even get to your second hand. I doubt that you will. With the free hand, count the number of times you say no to crises in a week. This will leave several fingers free. Use these free fingers to point people toward their own resolutions, after you have listened carefully and issued good advice and counsel.

10
Applied Time Management: The Pyramid of Proficiency

A Look at What You'll Learn:

- A model for applied efforts to become more efficient
- How to get control over what controls you
- How to improve the access to the things you need
- How to manage communication and save time

While self-management is clearly the most significant aspect of time management, we must also consider the work environment. Actually, I should say *environments*, given the multiple locations of work these days. If we assume that your self-management is based on balanced urgency-importance choices, we can begin to bring in outside variables that serve as opportunities to help prioritize your time as well as the time of others.

Every industry has its own set of work strategies that can be targets for increasing efficiency. An example in the technical trades would be *human factors*—that is, the ease with which machines or forms or technical procedures are used because of their design. The arrangement of the letters on a typewriter or computer keyboard is a good example of a technical human factors challenge. Many attempts have been made to rearrange the letters and punctuation marks in an effort to speed typing and reduce fatigue. In deciding on the exact location of the keys, several variables had to be studied: differences in digit flexibility, length of the reach, and the frequency of use of a letter needed to enter the most commonly entered words. In addition to these aspects, human factors engineers had to study mechanical aspects of the machines—such as returns, paper loading, centering, backspacing, tabbing, the chang-

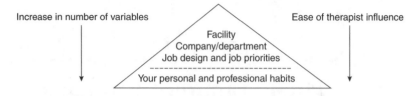

FIGURE 10-1. The pyramid of proficiency. In face 1, the ease of influence, the number of variables and ease with which a therapist-supervisor can influence efficiency measures increase as we move from facility issues toward personal and professional habits. This assumes that the therapist-supervisor is making concerted efforts to move toward a self-managed lifestyle.

ing of ribbons or cartridges—as well as the ergonomics such as the height of the computer screen and the reach to the keyboard itself. When all of these variables are optimally adjusted, efficiency is maximized.

The Three Faces of Ease

The rehabilitation world has its own esoteric set of efficiency variables. If you have developed an effective self-managed work style and have time to think about important things in a planned, nonurgent fashion, you can begin to attack some of these outside variables that eat up work time. I call this *applied* time management. In thinking about effort spent to control time, it is helpful to visualize a hierarchy of things over which you can have influence if you are a proficient manager. It is a concept I call the *pyramid of proficiency*. As a pyramid, it presents three triangular sides or faces, named *the three faces of ease*. Each face describes the ease with which an application of time management can be attained:

- Face 1 = Ease of influence

- Face 2 = Ease of access

- Face 3 = Ease of communication

Figure 10-1 shows face 1 of the pyramid, *the ease of influence*.

Face 1: Getting Control Over What Controls You

The influence we seek here is related to policies and procedures. Both the number of time-related variables and the ease with which you can influence these variables increase as you move from top to bottom. Note that the greatest influence is below the dotted line, in your personal and professional habits, because, ostensibly, you should have the most control over yourself. Those categories above the dotted line in this face represent the external policy and procedure (P&P) variables of the work environment that affect how you and your supervisees accomplish the work.

THE FACILITY

I use "facility" as a catch-all term for the schools, hospitals, nursing homes, outpatient clinics, group homes, ALCs, retirement homes, or private homes where you do your work. It could also represent a floor where you are placed within a hospital for which you work. In all of these work situations, there are policies, procedures, and expectations at the facility level that influence the use of your time. Some can be influenced by you, but most cannot. If you make the effort to study facility variables, you might find that *some* can be adjusted to change the shape of the events you need for stuffing your time box. The following is a list of possible facility variables that you might try to influence:

- Hours/days of service

- Mandatory meeting attendance requirements

- Supply/equipment ordering procedures

- Duplication of documentation

- Non–rehabilitation-related duties

- Insurance verification procedures

- Customer service responses

- Admission/skilling procedures

- Equipment repair strategies

I am sure that you can double or triple the length of this list if you spend some time thinking about it. The upshot of this discussion is that you must not assume that rules and regulations are sacrosanct. If they cramp time and efficiency, go after them. Just remember that if you are a visitor on someone else's turf, tread lightly.

COMPANY/DEPARTMENT

Many companies are beginning to retool. With reduced revenues and increased regulation, the industry cannot maintain the old model in which the therapist does the treatment with support from the assistants and techs. As one PT put it the other day, "It's the assistants and techs who will do the work now; we are merely treatment managers."

This is a hard pill to swallow, just as it was for the physicians in the late 1980s. You have to redirect some of your thinking and attempts to influence. If the company expects you to oversee a treatment team, you need additional support to accomplish that transition. That support might be in the form of computers with modems, keystroked logs, and other documentation, versus the traditional hand-written methods. It could also be assigning secretarial staff to therapists to assist with paperwork, mailing, and telephones. It might mean teaching you to use spreadsheets to compute daily productivity for predicting staff needs the next day. Could a van with a mat and some equipment be used to handle the rural treatment needs?

And what about forms? How often do you record the same information on three to four different forms on the same day? How much time is wasted there? Is there a "form committee" in your organization? Has the design of forms been reviewed within the past 2 years? Are you the person to suggest changes?

The list is endless, but the point is made. In terms of support from the company, part of *your* time management solution is *your* assertiveness. You can't sit back and be bombarded by changes in the industry and absorb it all as your personal problem. It is not business as usual out there. Insist on dialogue and offer to help re-engineer the company. That's part of being a responsible employee.

I doubt that I am any more of a rebel than you. I am not trying to create a revolution here, but I do dislike watching the days pile up on you until it's Saturday at noon, and you're doing Wednesday's progress notes on five patients. Your managers are probably scrambling right now to figure out how to respond to all of this turmoil and productivity pressure. They need your help. You are striving to find out what's efficient. You need their help. Take a deep breath, do your homework, walk in there, and ask, "Can we talk?" It may be that you can have *some* influence on your own company or department to help you become more efficient.

JOB DESIGN/JOB PRIORITIES

Often I hear the complaint, "This job is impossible." Well, maybe it is! Maybe it used to be the jobs of two people, but cutbacks brought it to you with one paycheck. Usually in this situation, you have at least three choices: (1) Request additional help or a restructuring of the position, (2) continue to be frustrated and inefficient, or (3) quit. One option is proactive, one is passive, and one is evasive; leaving the job merely puts you somewhere else, where the problems are not likely to be much different.

Jobs are not created by God. They are created by people. Sometimes people screw up and a job is ill designed. In fact, as middle management withers in the next few years, this is more likely to happen, because owners and administrators will become more distant from the work. Your job might be in need of analysis. Is it too big for one person? Too scattered across settings to allow you to be productive? Without sufficient reward to keep you motivated? One aspect of time management is figuring this out for yourself. Is the job actually a miscalculation on the part of management, or are you just the wrong person for this particular position? If you honestly feel that the former is true, write up an assessment of the needs (there are those clinical skills again!), and submit it for consideration. Don't sit and stew.

Job duties need to be prioritized. What are the priorities of your job? This is a big issue, because the answer is not at all clear for many therapists right now in this country. You are trained to be a therapist, but you are also a supervisor (although you are rarely *called* a supervisor). You are trained to be a therapist, but you are a politician. You are trained to be a therapist, but you are doing less therapy every day. What *is* this job anyway?

Ask! Most job descriptions are merely a list of duties and responsibilities, with credential and physical exertion requirements thrown in at the end; they rarely *prioritize* anything. Also, we have all of these add-ons, like team leader, site manager, clinical coordinator, or senior staff, which bring additional responsibilities that may or may not be in the basic job description. You have to figure out the critical mass of the job.

Ask! Is supervision the priority? Keeping the building happy? Doing evaluations and hands-on treatment? Chart reviews? Additional QA? Being a clinical expert for the discipline? Being a trainer? In-services? Keeping the case managers happy?

We know that prioritizing the roles of a therapist is simply not that simple, right? Needs change almost weekly, and by the time you've changed the job description, they change again. For this reason—this constant change in the work—it is imperative that you keep the issue of priorities in *your* job up front and personal with *your* manager. If you have regular discipline or management meetings, implore your leaders to keep you on top of the priorities. And don't fail to do the same for your own supervisees.

One final reminder on influence: The impact you can have on changing your facility, company or department, or job pales in comparison with what you do in changing yourself; if you are addicted to urgency, you will merely reshuffle a new deck.

Face 2: Ease of Access

As we move through a work day, we encounter dozens of situations in which time could be saved if we simply had better access to some-

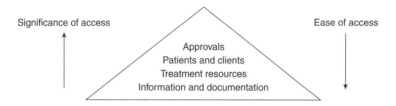

Significance of access

Ease of access

Approvals
Patients and clients
Treatment resources
Information and documentation

FIGURE 10-2. The pyramid of proficiency. In face 2, the ease of access is inversely related to the ease of significance as we move from "approvals" to "information and documentation." This reinforces the importance of developing vertical and horizontal relationships at many levels, because the most significant source of proficiency (approvals) must be wrested from other individuals, such as physicians, directors of nursing, and administrators.

thing we need. Obviously, barriers to access affect time usage and efficiency; such barriers are technical, procedural, or situational in nature. Thus, face 2 reflects a hierarchy I call the *ease of access*, as shown in Figure 10-2.

On this face, the *significance* of the access actually decreases as we move down toward the base of the pyramid. For example, without a required physician order to treat (an approval), you cannot access the patient or client, cannot use the supplies to treat, and have nothing to document until you have provided the skilled service. The *ease* of access, however, becomes greater as you move down from "approvals" to "information and documentation," because, again, these are generally things over which you have more control.

APPROVALS

The inability to access timely approvals or decisions is extremely frustrating for all staff. When we are blocked from moving forward with a patient or a project because a nurse, physician, or manager fails to act, our time efficiency is adversely affected. Items requiring approval—such as those shown in Table 10-1—cause us enormous headaches when a delay occurs. This is because of the "nondomino effect" they cause: Things simply don't unfurl.

Table 10-1. Items Requiring Approval

Patient screens
Evaluation and treatment orders
Order clarification
Equipment purchases
New supply items
New techniques
New staff hiring
Continuing education event attendance
Vacation request and coverage
New program installation
Contract signatures

Without an approval or decision, we cannot get our work done. We are often one or two parties away from influencing the *making* of the decision, and there is little that we can do to move the process along. If access to decisions was easy to accomplish, it would not be at the top of the pyramid. The best advice I can offer here is to carefully study "sentence blocking" in Part V, which deals with conflict resolution. Letting people know the exact consequences of their failure to make timely decisions or give needed approvals is, in the long run, a time-saving strategy. Also, if you can reduce the number of people between you and the source of the decision, you will have made a significant step forward in terms of empowerment and efficiency. Assert yourself without being aggressive or obnoxious.

PATIENTS AND CLIENTS

With regard to access to patients and clients, we see a new slant on applied time management. Here the issue is *too much time*, not insufficient time:

- Too much time spent with each patient or client (resulting in the inability to access *enough* clients or patients)

- Too much time spent unproductively for lack of access to *any* patients or clients (a census or volume problem)

Treatment time allocated to each visit has been alluded to several times, because the amount tends to be legislated by the method of reimbursement. You will recall the dilemma I cited earlier, when a company was attempting to shift from a unit-based economy to one based on a per-visit scheme; this was a classic example of a situation in which a manager could influence time usage and efficiency.

The use of concurrent treatments and care extenders have been effective methods of dealing with a high volume of patients for years. Here the problem is slightly different, because the therapist must spread his or her influence over several patients and staff at once. This requires the development of excellent instruction skills (for patients) and delegation skills (for staff), to maximize efficiency.

When a *lack of patients or clients* prevents access, we have a more difficult problem, because the sources of the problem are fairly remote. The reasons for low census or caseload could be many: poor image of the company, poor services, weak marketing, wrong niche, no reimbursement for services, poor physician relations, delays in verification of insurance, and many other things that would come under the ease-of-influence category. Therefore, beyond attempting to influence such patient/client supply variables, you might have to be proactive yourself in case-finding. The obvious activities here are increasing the number of screens, making calls for referrals, performing preadmission assessments, looking for new treatment niches, and so on. Even case-finding by walking around might be in order. Such are the tasks demanded by a changing landscape.

TREATMENT RESOURCES

Nothing gets a therapist going faster than the lack of access to treatment resources such as supplies, equipment, and DME. Such inaccessibility slows us down, makes us less productive, and makes us feel like something really *stupid* is happening right here in River City! And it is particularly embarrassing to have to explain to a patient, family member, nurse, or physician that you cannot proceed because a needed resource is held up somewhere for some unknown reason.

If a delay in shipping is the source of the problem, we feel fairly helpless. We all know the reasons for such delays (communication breakdowns, busy suppliers, back orders, wrong orders, etc.), and most of us just wait. However, we can improve access by suggesting a change in protocols or perhaps a change in the supplier. I have seen whole companies change the supplier because of the complaints of one persistent therapist. Sometimes it is a simple human factors problem, such as the design of the order form, so take action: Try to have the form changed. Make suggestions for that change.

The other access problem with treatment resources concerns control and location. If supplies, forms, or equipment that we need are under the jurisdiction of another discipline (nursing, billing, medical records, activities/TR, maintenance, etc.), they must be made to be accessible to *us*. I have seen this dilemma surface with wound-care supplies, and it can get ugly. A therapist comes in on the weekend or after hours, and the one person with the key to the supply cabinet is gone with no key in sight. The same is true with wheelchairs, activities of daily living (ADLs) supplies, thickening agents for feeding, and a host of other items that seem to end up behind locked doors.

The proximity of treatment resources is another area you might target to enhance efficiency. The location of the gym, modalities, and charting space are classic examples. I worked in one nursing home where the gym was two floors away from the Medicare wing, and at least 20 minutes were lost for every mat treatment because of the transporting of the patients. Because the gym was located in a converted patient room, all that was needed to increase efficiency was to trade out the rooms to get the gym within 5 minutes of the patients.

I once did a study of the charge-entering procedures at a hospital and found that everyone was crammed in on a half-dozen computer terminals at the same time when the day ended. This was marginally acceptable when the therapists were salaried, but it became a financial nightmare because of overtime when they became hourly. The solution: more terminals and scheduled versus random access.

Take the time *now* to sit down and work on these efficiency problems before valuable time is wasted and crises are created.

INFORMATION AND DOCUMENTATION

How often have you heard your employees complain about not being able to get enough information about a patient to proceed? Have there been times when you were blocked from moving ahead on a DME purchase for lack of knowledge about reimbursement? What about treatment and diagnosis codes for billing?

Information is the one thing we should be able to access quickly and efficiently. Timely patient documentation is required in all settings, yet considerable time is spent calling around, duplicating orders and treatments, and so on, when the necessary information is right there in the chart! Press your employees to read!

Too much documentation is an equally disturbing time management problem. For example, I once worked with a certified driving instructor who averaged about 17 pages of transcribed, single-spaced narrative in each of her evaluations. Besides wasting her own time and that of an hourly transcriber, she annoyed the physicians who had to wade through her verbiage to get to the signature line. She was replaced by a woman who hand-wrote the evaluations on a single page.

With the arrival of low-cost PCs, e-mail, faxing, scanning, inexpensive manuals, and widespread copier capability, you should be able to keep your employees (and yourself) well supplied with documentation resources. A blank spot on a form, where an ICD-9 or current procedural technology (CPT) code should have been entered, just means more work for someone else and more time lost. Left blank and submitted, it could mean a focused review.

Access to information about the facility, your company, the discipline(s), the industry, and health care in general is very important to employees. They work more efficiently when they feel well informed and spend less time around the proverbial water cooler

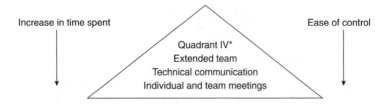

FIGURE 10-3. The pyramid of proficiency. Face 3, the ease of communication, reflects the effort to apply time management techniques to communication. In moving downward from nonwork-related chatter (quadrant IV* activities) to focused supervision (individual and team meetings), the supervisor should place more emphasis on control over the communication that occurs. (*From The Seven Habits of Highly Effective People. Copyright 1989 Stephen R. Covey. Reprinted with permission. All rights reserved.)

chewing on rumors if their fears are assuaged by honest, timely information. My motto has always been "Better a spoken pipeline than a whispered grapevine."

Face 3: Ease of Communication
The final face on the pyramid of proficiency deals with communication. Possibly the most overused word in the English language, *communication* gets blamed for everything from poor morale to bad breath. In the context of time management, I view communication as the glue that holds all other efforts together. If we cannot relay the information we have in an efficient manner, the quality of that information has little meaning or utility. The emphasis I placed on developing relationships in stage V of self-management techniques infers steady, solid communication, because that is what relationships are built on.

Let's take a look at face 3 (Figure 10-3) for its contribution to the overall hierarchy of applied time management.

Because we work in the service business, communication assumes an inordinate amount of our time. In working our way from top to bottom in face 3, we move from trying to curtail casual nonproductive chatter to streamlining face-to-face communication with our teams.

QUADRANT IV*

You will recall that *quadrant IV* refers to activities that are neither urgent nor important. In the current context—gaining time by managing communication—this represents those run-on personal conversations that eat up so much time. Casual discussions with other staff (both rehabilitation and nonrehabilitation) are important, because that is how relationships are strengthened, but you must keep them from getting out of hand. In your own conversations, you must role-model genuine interest that is balanced by the need to get things done. Employees like and want a humanistic supervisor, but they also respect the role you must play as a manager of time (and conversations). I would venture to guess that some of our employees spend as much as 20% of their days talking about nonwork-related topics. In my book (literally), that is a problem.

Unless you are hovering over such people, it is difficult to manage this time-consuming problem. Many of us have created checklists of nonbillable activities (NBA), such as meetings, travel, training, and so forth, in an effort to redirect behavior toward profitability. Invariably, there is a discrepancy of 2–4 hours between hours paid and hours reported on the NBA forms. These little pieces of data can prove useful in focusing on idle chatter as a reason for poor productivity.

EXTENDED TEAM

There are two areas to be discussed here: (1) improving communication within the extended team, and (2) reducing the number of meetings you or your team must attend.

Improving communication within an extended team is another great challenge for the time-conscious supervisor. Having good meeting-facilitation skills is certainly helpful, but many of these communication snafus happen when you are not even present. More frustrating yet is the situation in which you are a *member* of the group that is led by an ineffective leader and cannot do anything to enhance effi-

---

*From The Seven Habits of Highly Effective People. Copyright 1989 Stephen R. Covey. Reprinted with permission. All rights reserved.

ciency. We see this quite often as participants in rehabilitation-related meetings that are led by other rehabilitation personnel, nurses, case managers, QA specialists, teachers, or medical directors. The inefficiency emanates from such things as disorganization, lack of preparedness, failure to move the agenda along, lack of control, and lack of closure. If the leader feels in any way threatened by you, your suggestions for efficiency will most likely be met with speculation and defensiveness.

My first approach here would be to attempt *some* kind of private intervention in a soft, subtle manner to help the leader run more efficient meetings. If that doesn't work, you are left with several other options, including

- Role-modeling efficiency yourself as a participant

- Asking your supervisees to be economical with time at the meetings

- Reducing the number of rehabilitation staff at the meetings (if plausible)

- Suggesting a time limit to the meetings to enforce efficiency (using productivity requirements as the excuse)

The number of meetings we must attend has become a major time management problem in the 1990s. About 6 years ago, I overheard my son Devin (who was 6 at the time) talking to his best buddy on the telephone. The friend had asked where I worked. Devin answered, "At a meeting, I think!" Ever since that night, I have been more conscious about trying to control the number of meetings I attend.

About 4 years ago, I had a team of six in a 120-bed SNF that had traditionally generated productivity in the 70% range. Suddenly the numbers dropped to the high 50s for no apparent reason; the census was good, the case mix about the same, the team was intact, and there was no significant drop in orders from the physicians. I was reluctant to press too hard on my staff, because they seemed very busy and hassled. In an effort to discover the cause, the team leader used an NBA study of billable versus nonbillable time to see how facility meetings contributed to the problem. *Voilà!* It turned out that our company's focus on customer service had gotten the team into meetings that they had previously not attended regularly in the SNF: restraint reduction, marketing, department head, planning, wound rounds, and so forth. The team leader was able to negotiate a reduction in both the number of attendees at meetings as well as the amount of attendance time per meeting, and productivity returned to acceptable numbers. She asserted herself and solved the problem.

TECHNICAL COMMUNICATION

The reference here is to the electrophysical methods by which we communicate. With so many new innovations in telephone and computer technology, you should be able to effect improvements in time usage—by both yourself and your supervisees. For years we have used communication books and grease boards to stay in touch from shift to shift because . . . well, because we just did. Now a personal computer costing less than $1,000 can serve both purposes. Unlike a communication book, a computer is wired to the wall, and it won't get lost in the shuffle the way the communication book does just about every other day. When it comes to displaying patient assignments, a computer also has advantages over a grease board. You can save daily records to create a database for studying trends in the caseloads, discipline breakouts, census, payer mix, and so on.

E-mail between facilities or floors is extremely useful, because it can cut down on telephone tag and overhead pages. The same is true for voice mail, if it is checked regularly. In the age of information, it is ridiculous to have rehabilitation staff running or driving back and forth from decentralized work sites to a home office; the time and mileage costs incurred in a single year would pay for most computers and telephone systems three times over.

I have either created or contributed to an internal employee newsletter in every administrative position I have held. This is a great way to keep employees informed while establishing the tone you want for the organization. Even a small team can have such an instrument; you might want to call it the *Weekly Update* or something more creative. News on the industry, the company, new equipment, upcoming in-services, new employees, birthdays, meetings, and policy updates can flesh out a blank page quickly. It takes a little time (maybe less than you think) and is greatly appreciated by the employees.

INDIVIDUAL AND TEAM MEETINGS

The last area of communication management is the one over which you can issue the most control. We discussed individual supervision at length in Part II and will get to team meetings in the next section. Here are a few things to think about in seeking efficiency in these areas:

- In problem solving, try to discern the universality of the problem. If it is common to many people, save it for a team meeting instead of working it over several times in individual sessions.

- Avoid regimenting your individual or team meetings such that you meet every week without exception. If things are clicking and an individual or team is doing well, skip a meeting and use the time for some other purpose. I have had employees that required weekly meetings working on the same team as those who met with me on a monthly basis. Use your judgment.

- If you are not sure about the last suggestion, ask the team. Pull the group together the day before a regularly scheduled meeting and share your thoughts. If you are perceptive, you can pick up on the need for a meeting from the body language, even if a specific topic isn't mentioned.

- If you don't need an hour for a meeting, don't use an hour! Being efficient and getting through an agenda is a compliment, not a crime.

A time study focused on your own supervisory and team meetings might generate a few surprises. Meetings can creep up on you and dominate your time rather quickly.

Table 10-2. Three Faces of Ease

Face 1: Influence	Face 2: Access	Face 3: Communication
Facility	Approvals	Quadrant IV*
Company/department	Patients and clients	Extended team
Job design and job priorities	Treatment resources	Technical communication
Your personal/professional habits	Information and documentation	Individual and team meetings

*From The Seven Habits of Highly Effective People. Copyright 1989 Stephen R. Covey. Reprinted with permission. All rights reserved.

A Final Peek at the Pyramid

If you move up the ladder into positions with more supervisory and management responsibilities, time will become either your friend or your enemy. The pyramid of proficiency is most useful as an inventory, a tool you use periodically as needed. Table 10-2 looks at the three faces of ease side by side.

Don't let my use of the word *ease* lull you into thinking that proficiency is easily attained. It is hard work. And as I said earlier, the time-usage cycle becomes self-destructive if you never pull out of it long enough to manage yourself. And if you cannot manage yourself well, you can hardly expect to manage others.

MORSELS

The handling of paper is an enormous challenge to every professional. The more active you are, the more mail you get. The larger your span of control, the more the hard copy comes from both directions across the boundary you manage. In a business that mandates the constant documentation of what you do, memos, charts, and mail become paper enemies. Here are a few tips to keep your head above the pile:

- Make a concerted effort to touch a document or piece of mail only once. This is one of the best pieces of advice ever given on time management related to paperwork.

- If you must retouch, sort into three piles:
  1. Throwaways (toss it now)
  2. Priorities (do it now)
  3. For later action (within 48 hours)

- Try to eliminate the source of throwaways. Are you included on in-house mailing routes that are inappropriate? Are you on commercial mailing lists that have no relationship to your work? Can you remove yourself from these lists?

- As mentioned earlier, make an effort to streamline documentation and reduce the number of forms.

- Instead of reading professional material during work hours, take a lunch alone once a week and read while you are eating.

- If you are able to reserve "desk time," bunch your phone calls, and then bunch your paperwork; avoid doing both at once—it's inefficient! If necessary, make an appointment with yourself on your calendar, to force yourself to catch up.

- Avoid paper clips for bundling small groups of multiples; they can inadvertently grab on to other documents, causing hours of searching. Spring clamps hold firmly, preventing this problem.

- Learn to file efficiently, or get someone else to do it for you. Cluttered desks and countertops *always* result in lost time somewhere along the line.

- If paper (including chart documentation) becomes overwhelming and a serious source of stress, reduce the *stress* by planning time to reduce the *paperwork,* even if that time is on your own time. Put it down on your calendar. You will find that this simple act of planning will immediately reduce your blood pressure.

IV Meetings: Congregational Communication

Meetings! Meetings! Meetings! Will they ever end? I define a meeting as the congregation of three or more people assembled for the purpose of communicating about work. One-to-one sessions are considered to be supervision or individual coaching, and a group of more than 50 is either a speaking engagement or a mob scene. The dynamics of a true *meeting* are unique, and facilitation is a special skill, maybe even an art.

As you well know, a meeting can be a very inspiring event or a total drag. Much of the responsibility for the process and outcomes of meetings lies with the facilitator. If you are good, you will actually have people looking forward to your meetings. If you are weak, they will be looking backward, as they leave early with some under-the-breath excuse about child care.

As mentioned earlier, meeting management is an extension of time management. A good facilitator maximizes efficiency, because she or he saves *everyone* time with a quick-paced, to-the-point meeting. A poor facilitator wastes both time and credibility. Also, meetings need to be seen as opportunities to maximize communication. At times that communication will operate on both planes (i.e., vertically and horizontally) and in all directions; other times, it will be strictly vertical, strictly one-way. Learning to recognize the difference, planning around those differences, and then facilitating effectively is the skill list for this section.

I want you to take on meeting facilitation as a challenge. The industry needs it. Too many of us fail to use our imaginations in planning and conducting meetings, wrongly assuming that everyone hates every meeting. They only hate *most* meetings and for good reason: Most are boring at best. Running a good meeting is just as important as any other supervisory function, so let's roll up our sleeves and get going.

11
The Most Expensive Hour of the Day

A Look at What You'll Learn:

- Why meetings are so expensive to hold
- What most rehabilitation workers think about most meetings
- How to avoid total failure in your meetings
- Innovative openings: How to keep your attendees guessing

If you think about it, a meeting is the most expensive hour of the day. If it is *only* an hour, you're lucky; many meetings drag on forever and begin to lose their focus. With the exception of the patient care, rehabilitation, or Medicare meetings (or whatever your company/facility calls the weekly patient review meeting), revenue is not being generated. Bringing together a dozen therapists, assistants, and aides for an hour could cost as much as $250 in salary and benefits while failing to generate revenues of about $900 (if you figure an average of $75 per hour per employee). That is a chunk of change in any rehabilitation setting. Spread it out over a year, and we're talking $13,000 in expenses and nearly $47,000 in lost revenue. Net loss: $60,000!

What Rehabilitation Staff Say About Meetings
Over the years, I've asked people in our industry what they think about meetings in general. At first there is a dulling of the eyes as the various epithets are sorted out, and then they shrug, saying, "Oh, I don't know, most of them are pretty boring." The second most common response is a little more fierce, going something like this: "Meetings, I *hate* meetings! All we ever *do* is meet!"

Why do our people have such a problem with meetings? First, there seems to be a failure to state the purpose of many meetings.

Many therapists actually don't know why a meeting is occurring at times. This is particularly true of regularly scheduled staff meetings or facility-required meetings that must be attended by rehabilitation staff. Apparently there are times when no real agenda appears, and people are meeting for the purpose of meeting, because it's on the schedule. Hopefully your applied time management will eliminate this problem.

Another common complaint is about time management within the meeting. Many therapist-supervisors or therapist-managers (of formal title) are thrown into the leadership role without training or experience, and they simply cannot manage the agenda effectively, not to mention the people. "Nothing ever gets finished" is a familiar tune, along with, "never starting on time" and "never *finishing* on time." You have been there, you know what I am talking about.

The final collection of comments surrounds the "control" of the meeting. I prefer the term *facilitation*, as you may have noticed, because it connotes a process involving participation; control implies more of a one-way street. Common remarks include, "So-and-so runs the meetings, we just listen and take notes," or "It's not *our* meeting, it's *her* meeting. . . ." The ability to stimulate participants toward ownership in the success of your meetings is another extension of real empowerment.

The Boredom Factor

Aside from the specific issues mentioned above, there is the boredom factor. We are dealing with some pretty bright, creative people in this industry, and their threshold for entertainment is fairly high. If you walk into the same old meeting with the same old unimaginative agenda, you're going to get the same old comments, not to mention poor outcomes. If you are sparked and fired up, doing fun things, and generating a few laughs, it will eventually rub off. Much more on this will follow in Chapter 12.

Avoiding Total Failure

In a treatment episode, you rarely have a *total* failure, that is, a lack of any outcome. You might not help the patient attain the function or independence you intended, but a modicum of progress is usually made. The same is true with meetings. You can conduct a mediocre meeting and still avoid total failure if you at least seek closure on some items. Not everyone has an electric personality, and few of us have the time to bake cookies and generate lovely agendas on pretty pink paper. There have been times when I have had to just go for it, without so much as a handwritten agenda for my own use. That just happens at times—particularly when an unplanned meeting occurs. But *finishing* is essential. Rehabilitation staff look to the leader/facilitator to, if nothing else, get something real accomplished during the time spent. Even if it wasn't fun, people can say that it was worthwhile if progress was made.

You might find it useful to look at meetings as if they were expensive pieces of capital equipment. When I was in the hospital, requesting $50,000 for one of those computerized dynamos for the outpatient clinic, I projected revenues to estimate the return on investment (ROI) for the purchase. Taking the ROI mentality into meetings will spur you to plan and process efficiently and effectively, because you are spending money each time you meet.

MORSELS

If you want to "keep 'em comin'" to your gatherings, "keep 'em guessin'!" Plan little surprises to spruce up the beginning of meetings to get your team in the spirit. Here are a few ideas for you to consider from past meetings I have either attended or led myself:

- Bring (or have others bring) special treats, like bagels, seasonal fruit, cookies, and so on to get things started on a "sweet" note.

- Change the meeting place to break up the routine. Private homes, parks, restaurants, community centers, gyms, or libraries (if you have exclusive use) are good places to go, to avoid the "same old meeting room" syndrome.

- Invite a special guest or speaker. A local celebrity, a treatment graduate, a successful ex-employee, a local professor (from a therapy school), or an entrepreneur might bring fresh perspective that inspire you and your team to new heights.

- Look for things to celebrate at meetings. Beyond the obvious, like birthdays, holidays, and company anniversaries, there are an array of things to remember with food and drink: new contracts, goal achievement (e.g., meeting monthly/financial goals), completion of large projects (new program, etc.), and welcoming/saying good-bye to staff. However, take care to prevent these festivities from dominating your meetings.

Obviously, you want to do what feels comfortable and appropriate for you and your group. Create your own list and try to keep your team just a little off guard from meeting to meeting. When you notice that they expect that something interesting will happen each week, you know that your meeting has become something special!

12
Group Dynamics
and Meeting Facilitation

A Look at What You'll Learn:

- Why you need to learn group facilitation skills
- How to amplify your impact through group interaction
- How to recognize and use *process* in your meetings
- Classifications of meetings and outcomes
- Why a group's process needs cannot be denied
- Why you must stay within your skill boundaries as a group leader

Gaining the maximum ROI for time spent in a meeting takes great skill. If you are like most therapists, you learned your meeting skills in junior high, high school, church, or possibly college. If you did student council somewhere along that route, you learned Robert's Rules of Order and agendas and some basic voting procedures. Since then, it's been a sampling of regular meetings at work, plus a few committees and task forces of varying sizes. Most of the time, you have been a participant, not a leader.

Presto-change-o! You are now a supervisor-therapist, facing your first meeting as a leader. You have an assistant and two aides looking to you for guidance. If you're good, you could become team leader and have 12 people in your meetings next year. The program manager slot is next, and that position hosts 31 at the weekly meetings. Five years from now, you could be in a regional position, planning agendas for a presentation to 200. See how quickly it happens? One day you are meeting to coordinate the use of tech time on the unit, and the next, you're fielding questions about the new capital budget on behalf of corporate. What a leap!

The "Group Movement"

To make that leap, you must understand group dynamics. Most likely, the earliest experiential work in small groups came from the religious sector, in Bible studies. This was furthered by the arrival of Alcoholics Anonymous in the 1930s and 1940s, when peer support groups, using the 12-step method, attacked the growing problem of chemical dependency. Most of the empirical research, however, was done in the 1950s and 1960s, and it was clinical in nature. Known as *T-groups* in the East and *encounter groups* in the West, this movement had a powerful influence on the mental health field during a time when the exploration of interpersonal relationships was paramount. There was a strong "touchy-feely" component to be sure—particularly in the early days, circa 1970—and many people in the general public were turned off. The knowledge gained about the power of group interaction was valid, however, and it gradually spread from the clinical psychology domain into mainstream business. Many Ph.D. clinical psychologists became organizational consultants, because the same intra- and interpersonal problems that plagued their clients in the therapy chair affected the quality of work in business. And with their training in small group leadership, the psychologists were quick to recognize that business leaders possessed substantial deficits in their understanding of meeting behaviors. The business types ran meetings the way farmers ran tractors: Twist a key and expect the machine to perform. Thus what started out as evening therapy for recovering hippies in the 1960s has become basic training for meeting leaders in the 1990s.

Because all meetings involve group dynamics, I will use the word *group* interchangeably with the word *meeting* throughout the remainder of this section. And frankly, I hope you will begin to see your meetings as groups, because I believe that that slight change in lexicon will make you more successful as a facilitator.

Personal Evolution, Meeting Revelation

Being from the West Coast, I was an encounter group guy in the late 1960s. I still remember my first group, an evening affair held in a private home with a local college professor at the helm. As is typical of the genre, we were being trained as we "encountered." The facilitator-trainer would occasionally stop the group to discuss what had happened, while reviewing the actions of the facilitator for the edification of the participant-trainees. At the time, I was so caught up with my own self-discovery that I didn't realize the value of what I was learning. The oppressed cried out their guilt, the abused spewed their anger, the aggressors asserted their dominance, and the shy just watched in silent anguish until they were gently prompted to speak by our leader. The techniques were subtle, but the results were amazing: People got down to it and connected in ways they hadn't before. I *encountered* weekly for 6 months, finally graduating with some kind of certificate that I have long since lost.

During the 1970s, I washed along with the tide as the "group movement" came to social services and education. By that time, I was facilitating groups with students, police officers, probation officers, mental health workers, social workers, government officials, and, eventually, businessmen (in those days, they were, in fact, *men*). The emphasis was still on personal and interpersonal growth in the group itself, but occasionally some work-related issues would slip in—a team struggle here or a planning issue there—and we would digress into a brief business discussion before returning to our therapeutic journeys.

It wasn't until 1983, when I entered my graduate program in organizational and industrial psychology, that I realized the immeasurable value of group facilitation at work. I was a full 13 years into management by that time, had led hundreds of meetings, and yet I hadn't made a conscious connection between my group skills and my approach to meetings. What a wonderful revelation when I finally did! My encounter group experience took me far beyond the facilitation training that came with the graduate coursework, so I was ahead of the game when I graduated. It was then that I decided to begin teaching these skills to other managers.

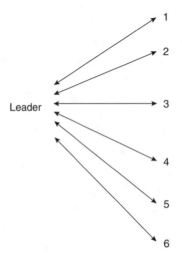

FIGURE 12-1. Leader in individual relationships with six people (one-to-one relationship). While individual supervisory sessions are critical to the development of relationships, they are inefficient in terms of time and the creation of interdependence within the team. Idea development and decision making in the absence of whole-team meetings are less dynamic because of the lack of active interchange among team members. (Adapted from DL Williamson. Group Power. Englewood Cliffs, NJ:

The Power of Numbers

In addition to being efficient, groups are *powerful*. In his book *Group Power*, David L. Williamson demonstrates this diagrammatically in a group of six participants. In essence, Williamson notes that a group of six has more power than the total of those six relationships would have acting independently in one-to-one relationships (dyads). Thus a leader meeting with six individuals, separately, would be diagrammed in a manner similar to that reflected in Figure 12-1. Because the leader meets independently with individuals, the interactive dynamics never occur.

In terms of potency, compare this one-to-one model with that for a *group* of six, as shown in Figure 12-2. Note that a total of 21 relationships result from the contact of one leader when 6 people are assembled for a group.

Even visually, the amount of energy portrayed by a group is far greater than the one-to-one situation. Groups provide more stimulation, more creativity, and more ideas because of the variety brought by the interaction.

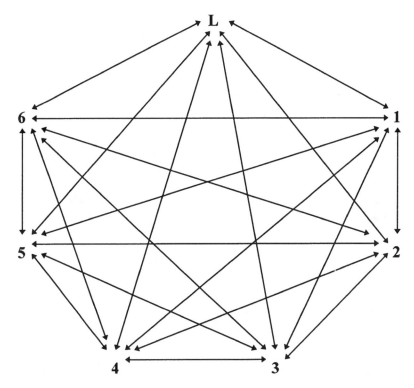

FIGURE 12-2. Relationships in a group of six. This graphic representation of a meeting reflects the potential power of multiperson interactions. In this case (a group of six plus a leader [L]), a 600% increase in the number of lines of communication is realized when it is compared with the situation shown in Figure 12-1, because the leader can access all six individuals at once. For communication among the other participants (i.e., beyond the leader), the number of possible lines of communication grows from 0 to 21. (Adapted from DL Williamson. Group Power. Englewood Cliffs, NJ: Prentice-Hall, 1982.)

It is important to note that groups promote personal and professional growth in people who do not ordinarily flourish in one-to-one relationships. By observing interaction among others in the group setting, hearing their ideas, and learning their methods of process, the more retiring employee can quietly gain from being a group participant. Such a person might not hit you over the head with it, but you can be guaranteed that she or he is learning.

Process Versus Content

Understanding small group dynamics is much like peeling the layers of an onion. Most group *leaders* fail to get beyond the dry brown skin of the group, because surface *content* (or meeting content, for our purposes) is familiar, safe territory, and the deeper group process is not. *Facilitators* are trained to recognize the layers and to begin peeling as soon as the gavel hits the table, knowing that in the lower layers lie greater participation, truth, understanding, and lasting results. It doesn't matter whether it's business or therapy, peeling rules apply equally.

Let's explore group process and meeting content a bit further. *Process* is the "how" of a meeting, whereas *content* is the "what." When you become process focused, you begin to key in on the dynamics of each member's participation and the group's overall interactivity, and you attempt to use those dynamics to better accomplish the goals of the meeting. Those who are unaware of group processes (or who are fearful of them) will usually charge on through a meeting with both eyes on one "what," failing to understand the "hows" of the meeting (most likely) as well as the "whys" (most assuredly!).

What exactly is meant by "process" when we are discussing meetings in the rehabilitation field? Consider the following categories:

- The level of participation (who speaks and how often, who doesn't speak)

- Leadership/followership (Is there a feeling of leadership or just wide open discussion? Is there a feeling of someone being in charge? Are there natural leaders in the group? Do participants know how to follow leadership?)

- How decisions are made (by consensus? by vote? by the leader? by the cliques?)

- Unspoken undercurrents (body language, glances and looks, awkward silences that make unspoken statements)

- Influential alliances (effects of friends, enemies, supervisor-supervisee relationships, etc.)

- Avoidance/denial/blaming (failure to deal with tough stuff; purposeful distractions/digressions; passive-aggressive behavior)
- Off-subject chatter (small talk, social talk, drifting away from topic)
- Role players (jokesters, enablers, rescuers, supporters, initiators, confronters, etc.)

Combine all of this activity with a full agenda in your mental food processor, and a simple meeting becomes a very complex event. One can, of course, become overly focused on process, such that nothing *but* process gets dealt with. This occurred frequently in the mid-1970s, to the point where it became nauseating at times, not to mention inefficient. For the most part, however, content will dominate process in the minds of most leaders of meetings. Many leaders view group process as a necessary evil and content as the quick road to profit. I could not disagree more, and once again, I plead for balance. Process is the *medium* through which you attack content effectively. You *can* learn to deal with process and content at once—it just takes practice.

Types of Group Meetings

There is no doubt that most of the meetings we have in rehabilitation would be classified as task-oriented groups. Some meetings—particularly those focused on team building—might be tilted toward process itself, but most are held for the purpose of attaining external goals. Take a look at Table 12-1, which offers a list of typical rehabilitation meetings, and see how it compares with your meeting life.

I may not have caught every meeting type on this list, but you get the idea. Some of these meetings will be highly content oriented, and some will lean more toward process. Given that many are held in combination with nonrehabilitation staff (nurses, social workers, etc.), you might be the leader, the co-leader, or just a participant.

Table 12-1. Typical Meetings in Rehabilitation

Immediate team
Extended team
Unit, floor, or wing
Patient/rehabilitation/Medicare
Utilization review
Discipline-specific
Scheduling
Restraint reduction
Wound care team
Special education team
Department head
Marketing/outreach
Regional
Special committee
Special task force
Training/education
General staff

Types of Outcomes

Meetings *always* have outcomes. Even the worst ones. To return from a meeting and report that nothing happened is to acknowledge the fact that you were disappointed in the outcome. That *disappointment,* unfortunately, is an outcome itself.

In being so results driven, we in business often fail to recognize that both positive and negative *process* outcomes occur in every meeting we facilitate, even if the ostensible *work task* is not accomplished. It is important to understand this on a personal level, because there will be times when you leave a meeting feeling depressed because no measurable results were gained, when in fact, several immeasurable things happened. The following is a list of possible end results from well-run rehabilitation meetings, along with a few challenges related to each.

- **Solutions to problems.** This, the most obvious of content-oriented results, is what most managers think of when they plan and conduct meetings. I have always said, "If there weren't problems, there wouldn't be managers," and meetings are where some problems—particularly those involving the whole team—should be dealt with. When a meeting is called specifically to solve a single problem or a set of related problems, it is especially crucial to be well prepared. *Challenge: To not become so problem focused that you ignore process, such as team members' fear of failing to find a solution.*

- **Planning.** In the proactive sense, some meetings (like strategic planning sessions) are solely for the purpose of planning, usually in the organizational development or marketing areas. Therapist-supervisors could be seeking roadmaps for program development, better relations with nursing, outreach for more patients, plans for additional staffing, and so on. *Challenge: To get something down on paper, even if it isn't finished; many times planning sessions become wide-open brainstorming brawls, with no charting, no notes, and no measurable results.*

- **Coordination.** This is a sister—albeit a milder sister—to problem solving. With shifting caseloads, additional work sites, requests to do off-site preadmission evaluations, and so on, coordination is becoming a regular outcome of team meetings. *Challenge: To invite participation and remain efficient; at times, it seems easier to dictate coordinative efforts.*

- **Improved interpersonal relations.** When groups solve problems together, there tends to be more cohesion, collaboration, and team spirit. Workers who are otherwise at odds are forced to put their differences aside and join the group process if the meeting is well facilitated. *Usually* (not always), this will result in improved interpersonal feelings, because participants are exposed to the thoughts and ways of someone with whom they would not otherwise interact. *Challenge: To avoid forcing teamwork and collaboration too early. Also, to avoid the temptation to promote love between enemies.*

- **Confidence in the meeting.** When you begin to feel the momentum of effective meetings and the results they can bring (along with a sense of what works for you as a facilitator), a certain confidence builds. Group members begin to expect certain strategies from you, and as meetings pass by, you expect certain reactions from them—the sum of the two yields an increased sense of purpose and teamwork. *Challenge: To continue challenging the group to grow and excel without becoming arrogant about it. If there are other teams nearby (inside or outside of rehabilitation), beware of the development of a superiority complex inside your group.*

- **Changes in the organization.** If you are very successful in your meetings, you will begin to see an impact in the overall organization. Beyond increased productivity and morale, you might start seeing other groups emulating what has happened in your meetings. Good meeting facilitation is effusive, and a great team stands out. *Challenge: To help other therapist-supervisors with their meetings without offending them.*

Process Happens

We're all familiar with the popular bumper sticker that acknowledges the inevitability of unwanted dung. The same is true with *process* in groups. It happens—because of you or in spite of you. *This is the first and fundamental lesson of group dynamics.* Process is like surging water behind a dam: You might be able to hold it back for awhile, but you *will* have to deal with it.

I saw a perfect example of this phenomenon in a private rehabilitation company that was experiencing rapid change. A highly significant (and popular) leader in the organization had left quite suddenly, and knowing that most of the remaining managers were feeling wounded and disoriented, the replacement leader decided to conduct a retreat the following week, for the purpose of strategic planning. The atmosphere in the office of this company was highly charged early in the week of the retreat. The management team was both angry and fearful, and morale was sinking by the minute.

In spite of my advice to the contrary, the new leader attempted to force his planning agenda on the group from the get-go. He had been warned about the inherent perils of doing this, the suggestion being that he instead allow some time for people to deal with their feelings. In no less than 10 minutes, the first emotional missile was launched by a manager who refused to ignore the obvious, and the group proceeded to process for about 3 hours. The replacement leader could not re-anchor the group around his agenda, because its members were not in a mental state to deal with his agenda. Roughly half of the original planning items were discussed, but serious damage had been done to the group's faith in its new leader. Moreover, it had been made clear that the new leadership model was one of "total task orientation." Neither the management team nor the organization recovered from this crisis, and they dispersed to other jobs in less than a year.

A few years ago, a well-known motor oil commercial espoused the value of regular lubrication when the actor-mechanic shrugged and sighed, "Pay me now, or pay me later." Such is the case with process. You might be able to deny, deflect, or otherwise contain it for a while, but sooner or later process will come out. This is true in supervision, team building, peer relationships, psychotherapy, and meetings. The smart leader recognizes this and honors it, particularly in groups, where process denied becomes process *amplified, stored, and biding its time.*

MORSELS

While gaining awareness about group process is vital to your success as a meeting facilitator, I must issue certain cautions. Participants who are experiencing personal crises or chronic mental health problems can unexpectedly lose their composure in a meeting that encourages process. Sometimes work is a haven for people who are hurting in this way, and their expectations are to bury their feelings in tasks for at least 8 hours a day while at work. Although rare, a simple warm-up exercise can evoke a strong emotional outburst from someone who is struggling to cope with personal issues. I once opened a workshop for educators with a nonthreatening warm-up I had used dozens of times before, and halfway around the circle, a woman went completely out of control in a matter of seconds. Responding to "What kind of animal do you feel like today?" she jumped to her feet and screamed, "I am *no* kind of animal today! I just want to die!" It took us about an hour to calm the woman down enough to get her to the emergency room for psychiatric evaluation. Clearly this fragile person was barely holding it together, and we don't expect to run into this situation every day. I want to make it clear to you that when I advocate group process and feelings and openness, I am speaking to human interaction for the purpose of accomplishing work in a work setting. I am not suggesting that you become an amateur psychologist who uses groups to fix the personal problems of your employees. If personal issues arise (as they often do), you must ascertain the level of severity and respond accordingly. This might mean using some meeting time to offer group support (in mild cases) or taking a break to get an emotional person to the proper resource for help (in more serious cases). Either way, stay within your capabilities and don't turn meetings into therapy sessions.

13
Creating Effective Meetings

A Look at What You'll Learn:

- How to select the best players to maximize meeting outcomes
- How to get the most out of the meeting agendas you create
- Why ground rules are important and how to use them
- How to set the proper tone for your meetings
- Group Facilitation 101: How to run an effective meeting
- When to use writing to support your meetings
- How to identify and deal with dysfunctional meeting members

The final parts of this section deal with the actual mechanics of planning, facilitating, and recording the outcomes of meetings. First we will look at you and some style issues and then get down to the logistics of actually *doing* the meeting. If you plan to continue your position as a therapist-supervisor, this information will be useful. If you are thinking about moving into middle or upper management, it will be critical—life as a titled manager is a life of meetings, and much of your efforts to be efficient will be focused on your skills as a creator of effective meetings.

Choose Members Carefully

Most of the time, the membership of your meeting will be dictated by design, that is, by virtue of the supervisory relationships you have. If you are a staff therapist, this will be the assistant(s) or aide(s) assigned to you. However, as you move up the line in management, you will occasionally be charged with assembling a committee or task force to complete a project. If it is a standing committee (e.g., QA, program development, salary and benefits), it will be a long-term group, and if it is a task force (e.g., organizational structure change, program development, marketing study), it will be short term. In either case, it is wise to spend some time thinking about the mix of meeting members.

There is an old management adage, the 80/20 principle, which asserts that a group is stronger and more creative if it is composed of 80% compliant members and 20% noncompliants. By constructing this internal diversity purposefully, you invite challenges to the ideas of the group from within. Discussions tend to be more thorough, and the stimulation level is higher. Compare this with groups that suffer from "think-sync," never stepping outside of the envelope to explore new approaches.

While I celebrate diversity in constructing my committees and task forces, I also avoid downright polarity. If I know that two people are arch enemies, I will avoid putting them in a group in which consensus is the norm. Conversely, I don't want strong allies with a known history of thinking alike to dominate a group as a twosome.

Unless representation from all sectors in the organization is required, I prefer a group of five or six for a task force or committee. With this number, I can move quickly while having sufficient numbers for brainstorming and accomplishing homework assignments. Also, the larger the group, the greater the scheduling challenge; finding a 2-hour block for a 15-member committee can be a nightmare.

The Almighty Agenda

There is something about a printed or written agenda that settles people into a meeting when it is handed out. Even if your meeting involves only two other people, and your time restraints dictate that you write it by hand, an agenda gets things started on a formal, organized note.

The content of an agenda can serve many purposes. Beyond a mere list of topics to discuss, an agenda can inform meeting participants of several other things, particularly if it is handed out in advance. A typical agenda for an outpatient clinic team meeting is shown in Figure 13-1. Assembling an agenda is an opportunity for you to be creative, so don't worry about the order of the items dur-

"Orthopedics Are Us"

Outpatient Team Meeting:
Friday, May 22, 1998
Clinic Conference Room, Noon

AGENDA

I.	Updates	Round Table
II.	1999 Equipment Purchases (tabled from last week)*	Tim
III.	Marketing Report	Sarah
IV.	Staffing Needs	Tim
V.	Upper Quadrant Program (progress report)	Cathy
VI.	Customer Complaint (Mr. Brockman)	Sarah
VII.	Company Picnic	Tim/Sarah
VIII.	Student Affiliation Program	Kelly
IX.	Other	?

Adjournment: 1:00 SHARP!

* Remember to bring your equipment request forms, complete with cost estimates!

This is potluck week . . . see sign-up sheet in employee lounge.

FIGURE 13-1. Typical meeting agenda. An effective agenda, when published, should not only reflect the content of the meeting but also the pertinent details of location, time, and extracurricular activities (such as food). Thoughtful planning, coupled with creative inclusions, can stimulate employees to want to attend regular meetings.

ing the draft stage. Just be sure that you have, somewhere, the following information:

- Date
- Beginning time
- Location
- Topics (and associated discussion leaders)
- Reminders of materials to bring
- Inclusion/exclusion of food
- Ending time

An agenda can also become an opportunity to stimulate participation and leadership. I have, in the past, posted or circulated blank agendas as an invitation for team members to contribute ideas or issues they wished to discuss. This can be done right up until the day before the meeting, as long as your time limits allow. If you have priorities that supersede members' contributions, do not request agenda items and then discard them.

Think carefully about the arrangement of your agenda in the final draft. If you are consistently failing to get through the list, cut back in the number of items. If you have a controversial item that you suspect will chill morale around the table, save it for last, so as not to lower energy for the entire meeting. Mix and match: Alternate announcements with discussions. Think ahead about keeping things moving along. Remember your creative beginnings and other surprises.

Most of the time, I list a final agenda item as "Other" and request last-minute contributions from the floor. The only exception to this is when the agenda is totally crammed or when the meeting is a single-item agenda (such as an educationally oriented meeting); even then, however, I will note that we can invite additional items to the table if they are deemed to be critical by the team. In so doing, I make it clear that this meeting is *our* meeting, not just *my* meeting.

Item-timed agendas can be useful or problematic. I generally use this approach—assigning a time limit to each agenda item—when I have an agenda full of many small topics to be presented by several different people. It helps to assign a timekeeper in this instance and to allow people to negotiate for more time on a consensual basis. If not accomplished quickly, this negotiating around time extension can become troublesome and annoying to the group, so be cautious about overdoing it. If it seems like a good idea to you, try it out for 2 or 3 weeks, and then do a perception check with the team to see if it feels good to them.

Housekeeping

Arranging for creature comforts adds a nice touch and shows that you care about your team members. It begins with choosing an appropriate place for the meeting. If you can escape telephones, visitors, and other distractions, that is ideal. Of course this isn't always possible, because we are so often relegated to some noisy corner in a hospital or nursing home where other staff, patients, family members, and maintenance workers are coming or going. I have conducted meetings in courtyards, at parks, in cafeterias, in gyms (many times!), and a myriad of other places to gain sanctuary from the hustle and bustle of medicine or education.

Be sure that everyone knows the location of the bathroom and, in most cases, that permission to leave is granted. Other comforts such as water, soft drinks, snacks, or telephone availability (advisedly) should be reviewed when initiating meetings in a new location.

The presence of food at a meeting has been a subject of some controversy. I personally like to have snacks—cookies, popcorn, fruit, and so on—because it furthers the humanization of a human activity. Potluck lunch meetings are also very nice, as long as the *food* doesn't become the dominant activity of the meeting. I have seen lunch meetings seriously compromised by the gathering and eating of food, not to mention the balancing of plates on the laps of people who cannot then take notes. It's your call. Set your expectations for the meeting and then design it to meet those goals; if you can set limits and get people to take their notes, go for it.

Ground Rules

At the risk of beating "expectations" to death, I will again testify to the value of alignment. When you begin meeting with a new group, a few minutes spent on ground rules will save you hours in the future. If you lean toward the democratic style of leadership, you might suggest that the group create its own set of ground rules. In any event, several important areas of agreement need to be established. For instance:

- **Purpose of the group.** Long or short term? Decision making or recommending? Internal or external focus? What are the expected outcomes? Will there be regular reports or one final report?

- **Promptness.** Begin on time, end on time. Establish peer pressure on this one, and you'll be glad you did! Remind people that lateness is a statement about one's respect for others' time.

- **Preparation.** If this is the type of meeting for which reference materials, in-between meeting assignments, or materials to be reviewed (e.g., charts in a QA meeting) are required, establish that expectation as a norm from the start.

- **Responsibility to notify.** If members are to be late or absent, are they to notify the facilitator or others? Are proxies required or accepted? If an expected report or presentation is going to be late, how much advance notice is expected? If one misses a meeting, is she or he expected to remain current by reading the minutes or talking to fellow team members?

- **Role assignments.** Is there to be a regular recorder or a rotating recorder? What about timekeepers? Will the leader do the redirecting, or can any group member suggest such movement?

- **Interruptions.** Do we take phone calls in this meeting? Do we leave for visitors? Do we interrupt each other or let people finish their statements? Can everyone agree to put their pagers on pulse as opposed to beep?

• **Negotiable items.** Can the group negotiate on the agenda? Can more time be negotiated on a particular item? Can extra meetings be added between those normally scheduled, if necessary?

• **Decision-making process.** Will the model for coming to decisions be consensual, democratic, or advisory to the leader? Will minority opinions be allowed in reports or presentations if there is disagreement?

• **Confidentiality.** Are all discussions confidential or only those so identified? How risk-laden is the information to be discussed?

Setting ground rules helps to establish you as a proactive, conscientious leader. In addition, by clarifying things, you can prevent the development of hard feelings later. For example, I have seen task forces that were created *only* for the purpose of making recommendations become disillusioned because their advice was not totally embraced by upper management. In each case, this occurred because the group had not discussed ground rules, and the members felt set-up by administration. The groups thought they had decision-making power when they did not, and they were resentful.

Setting the Tone of a Meeting

Imagine yourself sitting down to a meeting with several other peers on an acute rehabilitation team. Things have been tough lately. Two positions have just been cut, everyone is feeling stretched, and the computer is down, meaning that all service logs must be submitted manually. The program manager enters the room last and sits stiffly at the head of the table, tapping her pencil impatiently, as the group settles down. With a furrowed brow, she stares down at the agenda that has just been distributed and murmurs, "This is *not* going to be a fun meeting. I'm tired, and my numbers stink this week. They are going to be all over me if this team doesn't start producing better."

Boy, I can't wait to problem solve with this lady, can you?

As the leader, you carry the most responsibility for creating the proper atmosphere in a meeting you organized—particularly when the opening gun sounds. In a problem-solving congregation like the one above, you must rise above the fray, be mature, and be a leader. Because you are the leader, the attendees at your meetings watch every single thing you do, from your facial expressions to your use of language. They cue off of you and will either ally strongly (in a nonproductive manner) or shut down if your mood is too extreme. Your clothing, hair, posture, demeanor, response to questions, even what you eat and how you eat it are subjects of constant study, and the reaction is incorporated into the overall assessment that is being made of you by your team. The phenomenon is known as *management theater,* and whether we like it or not, it is a reality: You must watch how you act—especially in meetings, where perceptions are more precipitated.

Setting a nonthreatening atmosphere, as hard as it may be at times, is essential to problem-solving meetings. Looking frustrated, acting angry, and failing to make eye contact is bad enough, but beginning with a pessimistic opener like the one quoted from the above program manager is even worse. You must remember that most of our people don't want to be in the meeting in the first place, and trying to create a morguelike milieu is only going to drive them further away from active participation. If you, as the leader, cannot muster enough enthusiasm to attack the present problem, how do you expect them to behave?

You might consider the following openers when massaging a group toward a problem-solving mentality. We will use our acute rehabilitation program manager as a guinea pig by putting some alternative words in her mouth:

> *"Okay guys, we'd better get started. We have some real challenges facing us this week."*

> *"How do you guys want to handle this stuff? We have a number of issues to deal with on this agenda. What seems to be the priority?"*

"I'm feeling a little overwhelmed and need your help. How about if we go around the table for a minute and see how everyone else is doing. Let's limit it to 2 minutes apiece, okay?"

"Okay, we have about 2 hours' worth of problem solving to get to in an hour. I think the computer problem is the one thing we can do something about, so let's start with that."

"Are you guys feeling as pooped as I am? There have been a lot of disappointments this week, with our computer and the extra case-loads and everything, and I just want to take a moment to thank everyone. We can dig our way out of this, if we work together to find some new answers."

Notice the tone of these opening remarks? The neutrality? The program manager making these statements enters the meeting with the same slate of problems as the one who began pessimistically, but she frames them in more optimistic tones. She uses collegial terms that make the problems feel like *shared* problems, not *parent-speaking-to-child* problems. Note her use of the following terms:

- *we*

- *let's*

- *us*

- *ours*

This is "teamwork-bound terminology" that promotes feelings of common goals and common problems. Compare those words with the ones used by our crabby program manager:

- *not*

- *I*

- *my*

- *numbers stink*

- *they*

- *me*

Taken together, these words shift feelings toward the negative and toward the supervisor as the only responsible party. This is what I would call *antiempowerment language*. While the supervisor is, in fact, the responsible party, she is not helping herself or the team out of their dilemma by acting like a martyr. This choice of words reflects a choice of attitude, and that attitude is parental in nature and divisive. The team feels that it is working *for* the program manager rather than *with* her, and I submit that high-performance professionals do not do well with that dynamic. Professionals want to be challenged. They want their piece of the action, their share of the responsibility. Then when success does come, it only adds to the feeling of ownership in the task (and the company) and increases the feeling of personal empowerment.

I was once told about a manager who, under siege for her team's productivity, barked at them, "If I go down, you're going with me!" A real confidence builder, that remark! To this day, I still hear resentful comments from many people who sat at that meeting. They felt that this manager had taken all of the credit for the team when things were good, only to turn the tables and attack them when things were bad.

Setting the proper tone does not infer that you must be smiley-faced every time you face the team. There are times when a sober, even sad, demeanor is totally appropriate. For example, I once attended a meeting on the morning following the loss of an exceptionally popular manager; the young man had died on the operating table during surgery to repair a damaged heart valve. To have forced my meeting agenda with a happy face would have been a totally ludicrous act on my part. Instead, I allowed the tears to flow as we reminisced about our friend and colleague. Once the grieving diffused, we tended to a short list of tasks. I have seen similar situations following the termination of valuable employees, the loss of significant contracts, and company layoffs. You must put your ear to the ground and be willing to go with the flow when leading a meeting; to be a Pollyanna at the wrong time is to look like a fool.

Supervisor Spielberg

Once you have established the proper tone, you want to keep your meeting moving along fluidly. Much like a movie director, you open and close your scenes (agenda items) with the sensitivity of an artist. There are times in movie making when a scene just won't come together, so the director moves along to another scene, saving the first for a later shoot; that is a decision that must be made to keep an expensive acting ensemble moving. In your Spielbergesque role, you must occasionally table agenda items when the group gets bogged down. Few things will zap the energy from a meeting quicker than a run-on discussion that goes nowhere.

A number of group facilitation skills can assist in keeping a meeting lively and energized, and they are difficult to teach in a book. If you check with your local community college, university, or community mental health department, you might be able to find a class in which such skills are taught. Also, check the references I have listed for some great tips. In the meantime, here are a few of my favorites:

- **Redirection.** There are times when a facilitator must assert herself or himself to prevent undesirable turns in a discussion. In the case of a bog-down, the redirection could be to another subject, person, or approach. If the discussion begins to invade confidential or personal territory or other hurtful areas, a redirection on the part of the leader is totally appropriate. Lead-ins, such as "This is beginning to feel a little uncomfortable" or "We don't seem to be getting anywhere with this" are effective and nonthreatening. Probably the most uncomfortable redirect is the one that shuts down the "dominator" (see Dealing with Dysfunction), whose long-winded monologue has become boring, aggressive, or otherwise unproductive. I usually use something like, "Thanks, so-and-so; let's get a few additional ideas on this from the rest of the group," or "Okay, so-and-so has a lot of feelings about this subject! What about the rest of you guys?" A delicate maneuver, but one that is usually appreciated by the yawners.

• **Prompts.** Every group has its wallflowers. After a few meetings, you will have the patterns down and will want to bring out the quiet ones without embarrassing them. Specific techniques include

1. Beginning the meeting with a sharing session, requiring everyone to participate

2. Asking a specific question of a silent participant

3. Making note of body language and acknowledging verbally ("So-and-so, you look puzzled. Was that unclear to you?" or "That seems to have amused you. Want to share the humor with us?")

4. Speaking to the reticent group member privately, requesting more participation in the meetings

• **Humor.** Not everyone is a Billy Crystal or a Jay Leno. If we look hard enough, however, we can usually find something funny in most topics. Humor, when used appropriately in a meeting, is a valuable tool. It can break up somber discussions, it can help put things into perspective, and it is known to activate in the right brain and assist creativity. You know the therapeutic value of humor with patients and clients, so don't leave your funny bone in the clinic; your employees can use a little comic relief, and meetings are great places to bring it to them.

• **Clever moves.** Even though you labor long into the night to create a masterful agenda, things don't always go as planned. Last-minute additions to the agenda or new people can cause meetings to shift in undesirable ways, so you want to be on your toes to make clever moves. Here are a few things I've used to enliven dying meetings:

1. **Agenda-jump.** If you've gotten stuck in a series of problem-solving items and sense a slump, jump ahead to something

more exciting; don't be an automaton compelled to follow your own agenda.

2. **Take a break.** This is a great way to alter the energy and get blood flowing again.

3. **Make a physical change.** Stand up and begin recording ideas on a flip chart or grease board. Move people closer together if they are spread out. Suggest that the group go outside and meet in fresher air. Here's a really good one: Cause an accident! When I was trained in brief therapy in California, the psychologist-trainer actually admitted that he would occasionally knock over a cup of coffee or spill an ash tray (in an era gone by, thankfully!) to help move a stuck client off the dime. I tried this a couple of times, but only managed to soil the floor. Even so, it might work.

- **Anger.** I know, you can't believe it. Mr. Nice Guy finally shows his real colors, right? Well, anger is listed *last* here for a very good reason: It should be the last choice in your arsenal of facilitation maneuvers. When a group begins to break ground rules on a regular basis and all other efforts have failed, a little ire might be in order. Common examples of aberrant behavior include chronic tardiness, side-chatting during conversations, failure to focus and be serious about serious items, and going and coming inappropriately. I don't like what anger does to the group dynamics in the short run, but I respect what it will do for the overall process in the long run, when used sparingly.

The Written Word

In addition to the agenda, a number of meeting support items involve the written word. The type of written support chosen is dependent on the size of the group and its purpose.

Minutes

The taking of minutes is a prime example of such a decision. For a small team of three or four, minutes are not normally needed; expand that size to 12, and it becomes more important. The chances of multiple absentees increases, and one function of minutes is to inform those who missed the meeting. Also, for focused meetings, such as task forces and committees, minutes help to summarize reports and presentations and decisions made. Accreditation-related meetings such as QA or restraint reduction *require* formal minutes that are signed and kept on record.

Supplementary Reading

When a group has much to accomplish in little time, it is helpful to request between-meeting reading of supplementary materials such as books, articles, and monographs. If such reading is *critical* to the group's progress, make the reading requirement blatantly clear, stick to your guns, and bust people who fail to comply. As student body vice president in college, I was the chairman of the student senate, a group that was forced by time restraints to operate under strict "read-between-the-meetings" rules to accomplish informed voting at the weekly meetings. We experienced a serious problem one semester when several student senators began picking up their materials on the way in to the meetings, then reading and cramming during the vote discussions. After the third week of watching these wrinkled-brow voting sessions, I removed all materials—with the exception of the agendas—from all student senate mailboxes 10 minutes before the opening gavel. Several issues were tabled that day because of a lack of informed voters, and some severe reprimands were issued among student peers. The aberrant behavior was all but extinguished for the remainder of the semester.

Charting

I regularly bless the people who invented flip charts and grease boards. The ability to record cryptic summaries of ideas and concepts for a group is undeniably useful, and I recommend it highly. I have charted for groups as small as three and as large as 200. The only limitations are volume (of words) and visibility. It is pointless to chart long monologues for group members who are 50 yards from the writing, because it serves no purpose. On the other hand, when ideas are free flowing during a brainstorming session, charting is an excellent way to capture them.

My enthusiasm for the act of charting is only equaled by my disdain for poor charting *skills*. Here are a few guidelines for proper charting:

- *Print* in large, *readable* letters.

- If you can, purchase grid-lined flip charts to maintain vertical and horizontal alignment.

- Be cryptic, but don't create weird acronyms or abbreviations; they can be hard for a transcriber to decipher. Certain abbreviations such as Mgt (management), Admin (administration), Nrsg (Nursing), Mtg (meeting) are okay, as are the traditional therapy documentation techniques (Dx, Tx, D/C, AKA, etc.).

- Use two or more colors and alternate with each item; it makes it easier to distinguish ideas and topics.

- Try to face the group when taking ideas, and then chart; don't try to listen or talk with your back to the group.

- If you are charting in advance, apply stickies on the edge of the sheets to help you find certain items quickly.

- If you are moving through a list of items that has been precharted, begin with the page folded up over the first item and move down, item by item, using masking tape to hold the page up.

- When a page is completed, stick it to the wall with masking tape (if permissible) for easy reference; avoid flipping back to find earlier items and wasting time.

- Practice! Good charting technique is not just functional, it is impressive; you will gain additional respect from your group members for this skill!

If you absolutely cannot develop good charting skills, select a group member and develop the skills in that person. Good charts are invaluable.

Draft Documents
One of the most difficult and laborious challenges facing a task force or committee is the creation of a form or document. Whether it is a

policy, a new admission form, a mission statement, or a marketing piece, the work gets harder to do when additional minds are added to the process. The ideas get hung up in the exactitude of the writing, the process gets bogged down, and people begin to get restless and discouraged.

The key is to separate the *idea generation* process from the *writing* process. Using your newly found charting skills, conduct a brainstorming session on what you need and what you want. Don't worry about form, just go for the nuggets of content. If you get stalled, move on to the next item and keep the process energized until everything has been brainstormed at least once. Otherwise, right-brain thinking gets stalled by left-brain details, and you don't want that to happen.

Between meetings, create drafts from the charted brainstorms. If your writing skills leave something to be desired, grab *one* other person and have him or her help you. Two writers can be fairly efficient; three or more is problematic. Don't worry about offending the rest of the group. Just ask for their permission to take a stab at the draft, with the understanding that the words will probably be changed. Keep your ego out of it and give the group something to bounce off of at the next meeting. I did this once with a task force that had been working on a new performance appraisal form for nearly 18 months. By alternating brainstorming and bounce-off sessions, we completed the task in less than 2 months.

Memos

I guess many people equate memos with bad news or boredom, but I find them to be an effective method of communicating with moderate-to large-sized groups. I use memos for the usual purposes—notification/cancellation of meetings, updates, and so forth. But I also use them as cover notes to drafts and to poll group members on various things that I might want to know, such as suggestions for meeting days, times, and places; reactions to between-meeting writings; and so on. While memos are less personal than face-to-face meetings, there are times when they are quite effective and useful. Keep them short and to the point, and *do not* use them to deliver shocking or painful news; good judgment dictates that such emotionally based information must be presented in person to allow for the answering of questions and the processing of feelings.

Dealing with Dysfunction

After a few dozen meetings, you will begin to notice certain "characters" who disrupt your meetings. With all due respect to the 80/20 principle, there are some behaviors that are definite outliers when they become dysfunctional for the group. You might have some unpublishable words in your own mind for group saboteurs and, frankly, so do I. In any case, veteran group facilitators develop techniques over the years for dealing with these folks, and I thought I would share a few of my own. Each outlier type is followed by suggestions for *in-group* and *in-private* interventions.

- **Latecomers.** Remembering that this meeting is the most expensive hour of the day, we should have little tolerance for tardiness. In a word, being late is disrespectful.

  In-group: Begin the meeting on time. Penalize those who are late by moving forward with your agenda, making them catch up with others later. Remind everyone about the ground rules, and make your point.

  In-private: Make it clear that lateness is unacceptable, and make it a performance issue if necessary. Review self-management strategies, and offer assistance. This is a zero-tolerance issue, because it invades the entire group.

- **Dominators.** As referenced earlier, these are the folks who aggressively push their own agenda onto everyone else. They talk too much, too loud, or too forcefully, making it difficult for others to express their opinions.

  In-group: As mentioned earlier, attempt to redirect them or the discussion into new areas. Do not embarrass this type of person with a direct assault in the group—otherwise, there will be a payback.

In-private: When this becomes a chronic problem, it usually denotes an underlying insecurity, and a private session is required. Providing feedback will often do the job. Also, for people who are cooperative but unaware, I have set up secret signals (a wink, a scratch on the nose, etc.) to remind them to back off during a discussion.

· **Snipers.** A sniper is a group member who takes shots at the facilitator or other leader inappropriately. The tone is usually humorous or sarcastic, but rarely direct. Sniping is a passive-aggressive shot at the leader and causes the group to lose respect if not remedied.

In-group: This is a tough one. While snipers want attention in certain ways, they usually loathe the thought of being reprimanded in front of the group. I will, with a light touch, say something like, "Bob, did you have a comment on that?" and see how it flies, but I will avoid an all-out confrontation, deferring instead to private confrontation.

In-private: If you are patient enough to wait until the end of the group, bravo to you. I would grab (not literally, of course) a chronic offender at the close of a meeting and confront him or her right then. Sometimes there will be a total lack of awareness (most often when the sniping is humor oriented), but usually it will be denial. Make your case clearly and with consequences. You have a responsibility to run a meeting, this person is keeping that from happening effectively, and the behavior must stop. Point made, see you later.

· **Procrastinators.** Those who fail to produce a report or presentation for which they were responsible can cause a meeting to die quickly, especially if no advance notice has been given.

In-group: If group ground rules include advance notification, I would make a case of this in front of the group. I would also require a spontaneous update to help prevent future transgressions.

In-private: It is only fair to explain the impact of procrastination on the meeting to an irresponsible employee. This is particularly true in a task force situation, when the report/presentation constitutes a major portion of the agenda. With a frequent recidivist, I would make this a performance issue and would refrain from assigning similar responsibilities in the future.

- **Underminers.** Few things are more infuriating than having a group decision second-guessed by a member after the meeting has closed. This is another passive-aggressive technique used by those who fail to challenge a developing decision during a meeting (while acting as if they agree), only to try to undo it later.

  In-group: There is no intervention during the discussion, because the behavior has not yet occurred. It is important to stress the importance of full understanding and agreement during a discussion, as well as a review of the ground rules. If a true *consensus* is being sought, members need to understand that this means 100% support of the decision once it is made. Consensual decision making means that a decision is torn apart from every angle until everyone understands and agrees in toto.

  In-private: Were this a one-time incident, I would most likely handle it in the manner described in the group. For repetitive violations, I would make it clear that such behavior is destructive to the group process and erosive to trust, not to mention respect for the leader. If the violations were outright efforts to undermine my authority, I would use corrective action.

- **Documenters.** You may have been guilty of this one yourself. Documenters are those group members who bring clinical paperwork to meetings, spread out in front of God and everyone, and proceed to divide their attention between the agenda and progress notes. They will nod vigorously, pretend to be involved, and even look up occasionally to assure you of the depth of their understanding of what is going on. As sympathetic as I am to the current overload of documentation, I stop short of approving of this type of behavior.

In-group: A simple, polite request to "get into the meeting" usually does the trick. Sometimes a mere look is enough of a reminder for some folks.

In-private: For the chronic documenters, a review of self-management *and* documentation techniques might be in order, as well as a discussion about the purpose of clinical notes. How good is documentation done late and under these conditions?

Closure

A well-timed, well-run meeting ends with a quick wrap-up and summary of key decisions and plans. Remind people of any significant changes pertinent to the next meeting, and thank them for their contributions. A brief look at the topics or goals for the next meeting is helpful, if you have the time and information, to give the group a nice send-off.

Closure, Part Two

This closes this section. I hope that you have renewed respect for the power of meetings. The disdain people have for meetings in the industry has evolved over time and with good reason. Let us now commit to changing the most *expensive* hour of the day to the most *extensive* hour of the day!

MORSELS

Long before the term *empowerment* was in vogue, I worked with a remarkable group of five that took exceptional responsibility and ownership for team meetings. The weekly assemblages were, without a doubt, the most well-planned, power-packed, problem-gobbling events I have been a party to in my career, and as the supervisor, I gained greatly from the experience. The setting happened to be community mental health, but that makes no difference. Here are a few procedures that made this group and its meetings so special:

- The agenda was owned by everyone in the group. Items were contributed from Monday to Wednesday in preparation for the Thursday meeting; they were quickly prioritized when the meeting began. Each item was given a preliminary time limit, and a timekeeper was always assigned.

- The leadership of the group was rotated each week.

- There was always food present, but it was not allowed to dominate the meeting. Some meetings were held in private homes to escape the business phones.

- When the group was within 1 minute of the time limit, the timekeeper would issue a warning; extension of the time limit required a consensus of the group.

- There was a strict limit to the length of the meeting; rather than running over, additional meetings were scheduled to accommodate the need for continued discussions.

- Universal participation was mandated; reticent group members were busted (regularly) for not contributing.

- Celebration of victories—both personal and profess-ional—were regular and elaborate; this group knew how to have fun.

- There was considerable respect for right-brain (creative) activities, because the group knew that they would hasten left-brain outcomes.

- Cross-educating was the norm; anyone who went to a workshop or seminar was required to share all pertinent knowledge.

It takes a uniquely committed team to create a meeting milieu of this type. This particular team developed innovations that were years ahead of the field, and each person moved on to a successful career elsewhere. I doubt that any of them forgot this special opportunity to experience meetings at their best!

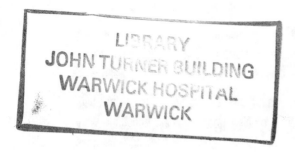

V

Confronting Conflict: Tools for Turmoil

The most prominent conflict facing the therapist-supervisor is the competition between patient care and supervision. Faced with this dual role, your inclination will be to treat first, supervise later, and live with the stress wrought by the discord. For the record, I want to state that I recognize this dilemma, that I sympathize with you, and that I have no magic resolution to offer. For the same record, however, I want to emphasize that the conflicts *around* you, if not dealt with properly, will only aggravate the internal strife you already feel. This section deals with that external conflict.

The ability to confront and deal with conflictual situations could well become the hallmark of success in the next century. In an industry so ripe with the potential to help other human beings, it is sad that we often hurt each other in the process of our respective struggles to do what we think is right. The scenarios in which we work are complex, the decisions are many, and the problems—as multivariate as they are now—will probably get worse in the coming decade.

In this final part, we first review the history that helps define the therapies and nursing, then review strategies for resolving conflict. My premise is that by understanding the nature of our differences as well as the commonality of our goals, we have baselines from which to better settle our differences.

14
Rehabilitation:
Teeming with Teams

A Look at What You'll Learn:

- Why it is critical to adopt a multidisciplinary attitude in rehabilitation

- A new way to think about team identity

- Why being true to your team is not always best

- The core team and multiple team memberships

I have always been impressed with the drive and determination of people who work in health care. The sheer will to be there for those in need, to solve the complex problems of anatomy and physiology gone haywire, and to absorb the constant loss of life and limb is nothing short of awesome in my mind. Unfortunately, however, that same fire for the work brings flame to the relationships that drive it, and as a result, we get disharmony.

Multiple Disciplines, Multiple Skills

Gazing across the world of work, it is difficult to find many professions that exceed physical rehabilitation for the sheer variety of people with whom we must work on a daily basis. While this statement might not be entirely accurate for the single-focus, solo-discipline clinic (such as an OT-only hand clinic), it is certainly the case in most hospital and long-term care environments, as well as in schools. In a typical 120-bed SNF, for example, a therapist could easily have multiple encounters in a single day with more than two dozen people. In addition to these multiple-contacts people, there is a host of others with whom one might have a *single* contact on any given day. Table 14-1 demonstrates the diversity of these groups, as well as the sheer volume.

Table 14-1. Daily Encounters in a Typical Skilled Nursing Facility

Multiple Daily Contacts	Single Daily Contacts
Patient	Physician
Supervisor (regional manager, etc.)	Family member
Assistant (supervisee)	Maintenance director
Aide (supervisee)	DME provider
Assistant (nonsupervisee)	Supply representative
Aide (nonsupervisee)	Pharmacist
Therapist (peer)	Respiratory therapist
Case manager (internal/utilization review)	Psychologist
Case manager (external/insurance)	Medical records personnel
Director of nursing	Building administrator
Assistant director of nursing	Marketing director
Charge nurse	Social worker
LPN/licensed vocational nurse (LVN)	
CNAs	
Wound care nurse	
Admissions coordinator	
Social worker	
Activities/TR specialist	

Given 20% variance and a caseload of eight patients, these lists predict that a typical therapist in a complex medical setting would have several hundred transactions with some 30–40 different people in a given day. Considering that most of the communication that deals with the essence of life—health—that is an astounding amount of human commerce. How do we keep it all straight? And is it any wonder that conflict arises with so many players involved?

A Different Type of Identity Crisis

It is a fact that rehabilitation is a team-based business. Few services are delivered by a single individual, and even when they are, there is often a family involved in a team effort to assure compliance on the part of the patient. One of the contributing factors to disunity in the contemporary scene is the difficulty we have with grasping team identity. Being human and naturally clanlike, we seek comfort in a work family that is recognizable, predictable, and small enough to wrap our trust around. In most cases, this would be the therapy team, that is, the therapist-assistant-aide ensemble in its various combinations. Thus, when a member mentions the *team*, the immediate reference is usually the therapistlike colleagues in the *core* team, and the identity is fairly constant.

In the more complex medical settings, however, the team expands to include CNAs, LPNs/LVNs, registered nurses (RNs), charge nurses, case managers, social workers, activities/TR specialists, and a physician or two, and the team identity gets expanded, if not confused. Now we are dealing with a half-dozen disciplines, perhaps a dozen or more perspectives, and a host of complications. Due to the numbers in their ranks, there are at least two smaller teams (i.e., therapy and nursing) within the greater team, and the propensity for bipartisanship increases. The ability to rise above your discipline to serve the greater cause (the patient) is a tremendous challenge in these large team situations, and we often see this challenge precipitated in weekly meetings. Leadership, cooperation, collaboration, and compromise are the operant skills critical to avoiding conflict. This is why so much emphasis was placed on group facilitation skills in Part IV—in the hope that as a leader *or* participant, you will strive to bring the right qualities to meetings. I would submit that it is also important to gain a better understanding of the history and perspective of other sub-teams (such as nursing) to be accepted members of the greater team. More on that in a moment.

Being True to Your Team (to a Point . . .)

This team thing can get mind-boggling. A couple of years ago, I was having a casual conversation with a PT who mentioned that the team was suffering from a drop in morale. We were talking in the office of a contract therapy company for whom she provided services in a single nursing home and several home-care companies. Because the nursing home consumed about three-fourths of her work time, I assumed that she was concerned about the therapy team (therapists, assistants, aides, etc.) in that facility. With a few questions, I came to realize that although she was actually on seven different teams, the morale problem rested with the six-person *wound care* team within the therapy company, not on the *therapy* team within the nursing facility. Because she consistently referred to "the team," in our discussion, it was obvious to her that the wound care team was her *core* team, and the remaining six teams were clearly of a secondary nature to her. When I counted all of her teams, they included the following:

- Company team (all contract therapists)
- Wound care team (her *core* team)
- Physical therapist team (discipline group)
- Home-care team (contract therapists doing home care)
- Nursing home therapy team (therapists, etc.)
- Nursing home rehabilitation team (extended team)
- Company wound team (specialized team of contract company)

Any SLP or OT could probably match this list, with a few minor changes because of discipline specialization. However, the point is made: Multiple identities/multiple allegiances equal potential conflict (both internal and external).

No one admires teams more than I do. The support, camaraderie, cross-training, socializing, and collective spirit that come with teamwork are near and dear to my heart. However, I have seen teams sabotage collaboration many times *because* of the strength of their identity. The wound care team I mentioned above was depressed because they had circled the wagons in defense of some protocols in which they had resolute confidence. Included in these protocols was an absolute 7-day-a-week treatment regimen: Wounds had to be seen by a PT every single day. The problem, unfortunately, was that a few SNF administrators and DONs had played musical chairs (as they so often do), and some didn't want 7-day coverage in their new facilities. The PTs bonded magnificently, dug in their heels, and sat back and watched one contract after another fall by the wayside.

I have spent a lifetime exalting the phrase, "Be true to your team!" The question now, however, is *which team?* That is something each of us has to decide for herself or himself. Just as I decided years ago that I am a husband and father who manages business (versus a *businessman*), you will have to decide if you are a team member who does rehabilitation, not just a therapist. It doesn't happen in isolation. You *need* these extended teams. Increasingly, in even the smallest clinic, your *core* team is just one circle in a series of concentric and intertwining circles that constitute the overall work team. Figure 14-1 presents a graphic representation of the various teams on which this therapist serves.

Remaining true to my physiologic training, I have placed a semi-permeable membrane around each team to emphasize the give-and-take that must occur between them. This osmotic attitude toward interdependent teams will go further in dealing with conflict than any post hoc interventions you may find later in this section. To function effectively, you will need to understand your own bonding behavior and make relationship decisions accordingly.

Bonding is one thing, but *bungling* is another. When a team becomes so stuck on itself that team identity supersedes common sense, we have a problem. The 7-day-a-week wound care example could be framed as partly ethical, partly procedural, because good wound care by a PT *should* be daily, and some would say that Medicare guidelines would demand it. At the time of this example, however, most contract therapy companies were not doing dailies, so the wound care team was somewhat outside of the norm. Furthermore, each wound care team member was part of an expanded therapy team in her or his assigned nursing home, and many were bucking the wishes of the larger group.

If you run down the therapy disciplines, you can generate a sizable list of other specialty teams that must function in a similar context, that is, as part of other teams. Table 14-2 lists examples of therapy teams that tend to be created by physical, occupational, and speech/language therapists. In virtually every rehabilitation setting, you will find that you will eventually become a member of several teams at once.

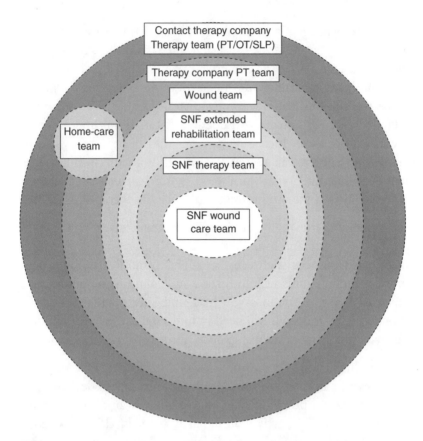

FIGURE 14-1. Multiple teams of one physical therapist. The combination of special skills, certifications, and facility or location assignments can cause therapists to become members of many teams at once in their daily work lives. Not shown in this figure is an additional responsibility for the therapist-supervisor: a management-related team (team leaders, facility supervisors, etc.).

The dilemma I have described here has no simple constructs, no definitive resolution. You must learn to flow from a tight peer group into a variety of other teams without undue bias toward outside attitudes. One way of doing that is to better understand your own peer disciplines and the major players in the other disciplines.

Table 14-2. Teams Created by Therapists

Wound care/skin care
Bed/wheelchair positioning
Dysphagia
Assistive technology
Dementia
Continence management
Burn
Spinal cord
Stroke
Brain injury
Cognitive
Ortho-med (bedside)
Hand/upper quadrant
Developmental disabilities
QA
Cardiac

MORSELS

A successful team is not necessarily a contented one. In fact, some of the most effective teams have suffered from notorious cases of internal discord. The Oakland Athletics of the mid-1970s was a classic example. The players on this team were forever fighting with each other off the field, causing sports wagerers to consistently bet against them in the big games—including the World Series. It was uncanny the way the A's would pull it together when those big games arrived. The players would hit the field, the chemistry would come together, and the focus was always there. The A's had all the right pieces in all the right places: power hitters, great fielders, excellent starters, and the best relievers of that era, not to mention top-notch coaches. Although the colorful personalities of the team dominated the sports commentaries of the day, it was the play on the field that dominated the box scores—and usually in the win column. I often think of the A's when conflict arises in a team, wondering how many hits and runs will be recorded in the final box score. Sometimes it is hard to remember that a strikeout is not a loss, it's just a strikeout, just one dent in the armor. Manageable conflict within a team can help to strengthen its resolve and fine-tune its purpose. So don't fear conflict; it is not your enemy.

15
Nursing and the Therapies: Key Relationships

A Look at What You'll Learn:

- Why it is important to respect professional heritage

- The history and landmark events of the nursing and therapy disciplines

- Why many nurses feel resentment toward therapists

- Why therapists often resent nursing staff

- How to help reconcile these resentments

Professional Heritage

On several occasions, I have alluded to potential conflicts between nurses and therapists. With humble trepidation, I take on this touchy subject, because I feel it is of critical importance to all of us. I know that I am bound to offend *someone* in the process, so I apologize in advance. I have worked with the four disciplines that are most closely associated with physical rehabilitation—occupational, physical, and speech/language therapies and nursing—and have immense respect for what is brought to the table by each. As a "No-T" (nontherapist), I feel I am a fairly objective observer, and I only want to advance the cause by enhancing mutual understanding within the professions. If this, in turn, promotes better teamwork and brings about less conflict, I have accomplished my goals.

Why do nurses and therapists have such a time of it? What fundamental differences are there—both past and present—that cause us to get caught up in the conflict and lose sight of the healing? Why do the disciplines go after each other behind closed doors? Why does alienation surface so quickly, so easily?

Let's start with a review of professional heritage. Through interviews and reading, I have come to know the origins of the four disciplines and want to share a glimpse of history with you. You might be surprised at what you learn about the disciplines, which I discuss in alphabetical order.

Nursing

Nursing has a history so vast that even the historians cannot agree on definite origins. The Latin roots *nutrix* (nursing mother) and *nutrire* (suckles and nourishes) immediately associate nursing with birth, motherhood, nurturing, and, of course, women. The profession is, in fact, dominated by women (approximately 95%), but the art and science of nursing go far beyond maternal instincts. In fact, it is interesting that Florence Nightingale, the ostensible icon of nursing, was not at all the motherlike figure that we laypeople would have her be. As an astute statistician, Ms. Nightingale almost single-handedly reduced British military hospital deaths by 20% during the Crimean War (1851–1855) by keeping meticulous records on epidemiology. Also, unlike her peers in that era, she was of upper-class birth and had to fight with her own family to be the nurse she was destined to become. A stalwart leader in public health, sanitation, and nursing education, she changed the course of medical history. What a wonderful role model for the thousands of nurses who have followed.

Finding a single definition of nursing is literally impossible, because the profession and its application are so broad. One clever saying is that medicine is the *cure* whereas nursing is the *care*. Another, taken from M.P. Donahue's *Nursing: The First Art*, defines nursing this way:

> *From the dawn of civilization, evidence prevails to support the premise that nurturing has been essential to the preservation of life. Survival of the human race, therefore, is inextricably intertwined with the development of nursing.*

The ancient cultures (pre-Christ) developed medicine as a science and profession but did little to establish a foundation for nursing. The first continuity came with Christianity as a direct result of Jesus' teachings of love and charity for the poor, enslaved, widowed, aged, and orphaned. The first organized nurselike activity came from the Eastern Christian churches and their deaconess movement. The widows and daughters of Roman officials—women of breeding, culture, wealth, and position—performed "works of mercy" by caring for the sick and injured among the poor. Nursing's first heroine, Phoebe, was a deaconess who took care of Paul and carried his messages; she is thought to be the first visiting nurse.

In the centuries following Jesus' death, the Order of Widows and Order of Virgins joined the deaconesses in spreading nursing services westward from Rome, finally reaching England in the 800s. Thus it is said that the first nurses were wives, widows, and virgins. Hundreds of hospitals were built during this era, and the first real nursing schools were created.

Unfortunately, the Crusades came along shortly thereafter (1096–1291) and wiped out the deaconess movement. What is interesting about this period is that military nursing orders evolved, and they often required protection while doing their work. One order, the Knights of Hospitallers of St. John, required that the nurse-nuns wear suits of armor under their habits. These particular habits bore the Maltese cross, which later became the part of the badge for the Nightingale Training School in the late 1800s.

The Reformation (sixteenth century) was a serious setback to nursing, because women were once again subordinated to men. Hospital work became relegated to "uncommon" women, such as prostitutes, prisoners, and the poor. In fact, nurses was considered to be the most menial of servants. This period is known today as the dark age of nursing.

The antecedents to American nursing came from Britain and the Nightingale Training Schools. The Nightingale model came to the United States in 1849 when a pastor and four deaconesses assumed responsibility for the Pittsburgh Infirmary, which was the first

Protestant hospital in the United States. Eleven years later, the Civil War broke out, serving as a catalyst for moving women from the home into nursing, where they volunteered in hospitals, infirmaries, and the battlefields. Dorothea Dix, already well known for her concern for the mentally ill, was appointed superintendent of women nurses for the Union Army. Clara Barton, who served as a tireless volunteer during the war, was instrumental in founding the American Red Cross in 1882.

The first Nightingale-like schools were established in Bellevue, New York; New Haven, Connecticut; and Boston, Massachusetts. Soon physicians and hospital administrators (who were also physicians) recognized the benefit of free services from "pupil nurses," and by 1900 there were 432 nursing schools in the United States.

The development of professionalism in nursing came in the mid-1890s, when the superintendents of nurses became concerned about the widespread use of untrained nurses in medical settings. At the time, the U.S. Census Bureau estimated that there were 109,000 untrained nurses and midwives competing with 12,000 graduate nurses. Therefore, they formed the Nurses Association Alumnae of the United States and Canada in 1896; the group was renamed the American Nurses Association (ANA) in 1912, and the ANA remains a powerful force in the health care industry. The formation of the original association was quickly followed by a national plan for the registration of trained nurses.

As you will soon see with OTs, the Spanish-American and First World wars helped establish the need for medical support personnel in both military and civilian life in the early part of the twentieth century. The first university nursing program was started at the University of Minnesota in 1909. In 1920, a Rockefeller Foundation study produced the *Goldmark Report,* which recommended that schools of nursing be independent of hospitals and that students no longer be exploited as cheap labor. Several additional university schools of nursing were opened shortly thereafter.

Table 15-1. The Formal Degrees of Nursing

Degree or Type of License	Year/Era	Location of Training
BSN	1909	4-year colleges/universities
LVN/LPN	1942	Vocational/technical schools
RN	1952	Junior/community colleges or 4-year colleges/universities
MSN (MN, MS, MA)	Late 1950s	4-year colleges/universities
PhD (DSN, DNS, DNSc, EdD)	Early 1960s	Universities

The nursing industry declined during the Great Depression, and hospital fortunes followed the same path until the advent of Blue Cross in 1937. As the first prepaid health insurance in the United States, Blue Cross brought the *hospitals* back, but nursing continued to fall, as some 570 training programs closed during the 1930s. Nurses were replaced by low-wage, untrained personnel for a while, until desperate graduate nurses came back to work for minimum wage. Because the professional nurses were not as compliant as their untrained predecessors and demanded higher pay, the relationship between nursing and hospital administrators never really took, and an uneasy alliance was created. Unfortunately for the profession, modern trends for nursing were set during this period under these conditions. As historian Susan Reverby noted, hospital administrators offered graduate nurses "low pay, long hours, split shifts, authoritarian supervision, and rigid rules" (Donahue, 1985).

World War II brought another increase in the demand for nurses. The Cadet Nurse Corps, established in 1943, sponsored nursing education for thousands of young people, who agreed to engage in nursing for the duration of the war.

Modern nurses are involved in not only patient care, but administration, research, and advisory capacities worldwide. Table 15-1 reflects the various degrees available to nurses, along with the year of advent and the location of the training.

Advanced practice nurses (APNs) have a specialized body of knowledge and expanded practice skills acquired through study at the graduate level. Some of the APN specialties are as follows:

- Certified nurse midwives (CNMAs)
- Certified RN anesthetists (CRNAs)
- Clinical nurse specialists (CNSs)
- Nurse practitioners (NPs)

A couple of nursing specialties are of particular importance to therapists. The certified rehabilitation registered nurse (CRRN) should be a therapist's best friend. A crucial player in acute rehabilitation units in hospitals and some subacute units and SNFs, the CRRN is the most experienced of the nurses in medical rehabilitation and must pass a rigorous exam to become certified. Having a full compliment of CRRNs in a rehabilitation unit is a luxury for therapists, because these nurses are more aware of the treatments and modalities than the average physician.

The certified enterostomal therapy nurse (CETN or ET nurse) has become increasingly important to therapists as wound care has become a significant part of rehabilitation. Trained in ostomy, wound care, and incontinence management, the ET works in several domains that directly affect therapy. The movement toward moist wound management is credited to ETs, who, along with key physicians, have also led the fight to remove cytotoxic agents (such as povidone-iodine [Betadine]) from wound care treatment. On the incontinence front, many ETs have teamed up with PTs to provide a powerful one-two punch, using patient education, nutritional adjustment, and biofeedback-based muscular re-education. Also, ostomies can be a major problem (both clinically and financially), and ETs are the best resource for therapists, physicians, and other nurses.

It is obvious that the struggle for acceptance has been long and arduous for the nursing profession. Their heritage is one of 2,000 years of advances and declines, with proper recognition having come only in the last 60 years. Still, given the dedication and commitment nurses bring to their patients, they remain undercompensated when compared with the therapies.

Occupational Therapy

Ask your generic health care worker what he or she knows about OT, and some funny things come out: arts and crafts; above the waist only; started in psych; all women, no men; they show up in clothes that are halfway between what PT and speech wears. Great mythology, but only half-truths (except for the clothes!).

Although the concept of "occupation activity" goes all the way back to the ancient Greeks, the roots of OT in the United States are traced to the late eighteenth century. The work *was* in the mental health arena, with the thought that the health of individuals was influenced by "the use of muscles and mind together in games, exercise, and handicraft, as well as in work" (Hopkins and Smith, 1978). This philosophy became the basis of work, exercise, and play as the modalities of treatment in modern occupational therapy.

The early history of OT is much like that of other medical disciplines in that its prominence fluctuated with the arrival and departure of American wars. After rising during the prerevolutionary years, OT-like work flourished for about 100 years, before dropping off for 25 years just after the Civil War. In 1892, interest was revitalized by landmark work done by Adolf and Mary Meyer, a physician and social worker, respectively. Stressing such ideas as "rhythms of life" and "doing and practice," the Meyers promoted wholesome living as a basis for "wholesome thinking, feeling, and interest." Thus OT-like work was moved forward in medical thinking by blending productive activities and recreation to emulate work and pleasure.

The first bona fide OT was actually a *nurse* named Susan Tracy. Working with the mentally ill as director of the Training School for Nurses in Boston, Tracy developed the first systematic training course in occupation in 1906 to prepare instructors for teaching patient activities. In 1910, Tracy published the first book on occupations titled *Studies in Invalid Occupations: A Manual for Nurses and Attendants.*

During the next decade, several key players moved the field toward new horizons as social workers, kindergarten teachers, and crafts teachers joined the ranks. In 1914, a layman architect named George Edward Barton actually coined the title "occupational therapist," stating that the fundamental principle of the discipline was "Not the making of an object, but the making of a man."

In 1917, the National Society for the Promotion of Occupational Therapy was founded, becoming the American Occupational Therapy Association (AOTA) in 1920. The AOTA remains the professional association today with some 55,000 members.

The expansion of the treatment into *physical* dysfunction began during World War I, when the job classification of "reconstruction aides" was created by the armed services to deal with the thousands of soldiers wounded in battle. During this era, the earliest prototypes of adaptive equipment and devices for measuring strength and range of motion were developed. As was the case after the Civil War, however, the field dropped back once again in the postwar era.

The recovery from World War II helped to bring rehabilitation into the modern era, as new drugs and improved medical treatment allowed for the survival of a broader population requiring occupational therapy. OTs diversified and became specialized in the treatment of certain types of disabilities such as peripheral nerve injuries and amputations. During this period, ADLs were developed, along with work simplification, rehabilitation for the handicapped homemaker, and training in the use of upper extremity prostheses. The first textbook written and edited by OTs in the United States was published in 1947 by Willard and Spackman, *Occupational Therapy*, and it continues to be a classic in the field.

In the 1950s, OT became an exact science, as the United States moved through another of many polio epidemics and specialization was further advanced. The treatment of chronic conditions such as arthritis, heart disease, stroke, and congenital disease (e.g., cerebral palsy) was added to the OT agenda during this time, and the Korean and Vietnam wars helped move the field further into the treatment of traumatic injury.

During its century of growth in the medical field, OT never left the mental health front. In keeping with the rest of the psychiatric profession, OTs followed the shift toward the social adaptation of the patient and the return to family and community that took place in the 1960s and 1970s. Today, OT is a very prominent player on the floors of this country's mental health institutions.

The growth of special education in the schools rounds out the overall picture of OT, which is now an accepted profession in the medical, mental health, and educational fields. The greatest numbers, of course, are in medicine—increasingly so in the geriatric arena—with the advent of Medicare in 1965 and the aging of the American population. Both Medicare and commercial insurance began to recognize the efficacy of OT in the late 1980s, allowing the field to train even greater numbers of therapists in the 1990s.

There are several degree opportunities in the field of occupational therapy. The technical education programs grant an associate degree as preparation for certification as a COTA. Three levels of professional programs are offered—baccalaureate, postbaccalaureate certification, and master's degrees—to prepare a person to become a registered occupational therapist (OTR).

It has been a rewarding journey for the professionals who have nurtured this discipline from "occupation activities" to contemporary occupational therapy, which, by the way, is not limited to treatment "above the waist." While the origins of occupational and physical therapy are similar, autonomy for OTs has been a bit slower to develop than autonomy for PTs. And, by the way, it is a bit frustrating for OTs and SLPs when someone is insensitive enough to post the sign PHYSICAL THERAPY on the front door of the rehabilitation department. Again, this is probably more reflective of the early acceptance of PT by other health-care providers than it is a slam on OT or SLP.

Physical Therapy

Physical therapy has been called the *oldest method of medical treatment*. The use of hot sand and rocks to treat pulled muscles and arthritis dates back to the Stone Age, as does the use of running water to aid the healing of infected wounds. The use of heat and cold to treat a myriad of ailments is documented in ancient Greek, Roman, Persian, and Russian history, as would-be PTs unknowingly made use of vasoconstriction and vasodilation to aid their primitive treatments. Although hydrotherapy was widely used by many cultures, it was the Romans who first made extensive use of public baths and sweat houses to aid health. The Romans were also the first to use underwater exercises in warm springs to treat the paralysis from war wounds and aging in the general population. Modern electrical stimulation and ultrasound treatments had their precursors in ancient times as well, when amber (rubbed vigorously) and electric eels and electric catfish were applied to treat arthritic joints and other physical ailments.

The therapeutic value of massage and exercise in combination can be documented as far back as 3000 BC in Chinese and Japanese cultures. And, of course, it was the Chinese who discovered and developed acupuncture as a treatment for disease and pain. The Hindus were known to be the first to specifically use *therapeutic* exercises, and modern Indians continue to use yoga to cure physical and mental illnesses. Both massage and therapeutic exercise continued to develop in Western Europe during the eighteenth and nineteenth centuries, with the most substantial contributions to the science coming from Sweden and Switzerland.

By the end of the nineteenth century, the early practitioners of physical therapy began to specialize. In Britain, physician *orthope-*

dists evolved, using heat, massage, and therapeutic exercise to treat problems with the bones, joints, and muscles. When these approaches became too time-consuming, the orthopedists trained young female physical education graduates to direct the special corrective exercises of orthopedic patients.

The polio epidemic of 1915–1917 caused a physician named Robert Lovett from Vermont to duplicate the British approach in the United States. He trained two women in muscular re-education for the treatment of infantile paralysis.

In 1916, Walter Reed Hospital in Washington, D.C., established the first physical therapy department. As would be the case around the country for years, the PT area was stuck in the basement in two small rooms, causing much of the treatment to be performed at bedside.

Along came World War I and the birth of the Women's Auxiliary Aides, which functioned under the Division of Orthopedic Surgery. Muscular re-education and physical training were not a part of the nursing, medical, or surgical care at the time, so the auxiliary assumed the responsibility for this phase of caring for the wounded. As the casualties began to arrive in the United States, new schools of physical therapy were quickly added, their graduates joining the OTs as reconstruction aides (RAs). It was in one of these schools—Reed College in Eugene, Oregon—where an outstanding leader, Mary McMillan, helped foster the progress of physical therapy as a profession. Reed joined 13 other schools in producing 800 RAs, 300 of whom served overseas as civilians. They were all women and mostly PE teachers before the war. As civilians, the RAs were required to follow all of the rules of the military during the war, but received none of the military benefits.

As did OT, PT dropped off after the war, because civilian practices were not yet ready for the new profession. However, Mary McMillan joined Dr. Frank Granger in codirecting a course of study at Harvard Medical School emphasizing electrophysics, electrotherapy, and muscle re-education. In 1921, 245 of the RAs gathered in New York City and formed the American Women's Physical Therapeutic Association, electing Mary McMillan as its first president. A year later, men were included in the group, which changed its name to the American Physiotherapy Association (the original name for the American Physical Therapy Association [APTA]).

By 1940, the American Medical Association (AMA) had established a Council on Physical Therapy, thereby giving its blessing to the inclusion of courses to be given through medical schools. Sixteen schools were graduating 135 students a year, and approximately 1,000 PTs were practicing by the time the United States entered World War II. This time, however, Congress declared that PT graduates would receive the rank of second lieutenant, qualifying them for commissions in the Women Appointed for Voluntary Emergency Service (WAVES). Some 800 of the 1,600 WAVES PTs served overseas in the army.

The nation's recovery from the war, another polio epidemic (1944), and a surge of industrial accidents in the defense plants spurred PT on to further acceptance by the public. Baccalaureate programs were common by this time, and graduate programs were in the works. The APTA recently celebrated its seventy-fifth anniversary, with membership in excess of 60,000. It is estimated that there are more than 160,000 PTs in the world, most of them in Western Europe and the United States.

Degree programs for PT are similar to those for OT. An associate degree provides for potential certification as a PTA, while baccalaureates and master's degrees prepare for licensing as PTs. The most encompassing definition of physical therapy comes from Ms. Thelma Holmes, associate professor in the physical therapy curriculum at the University of Florida (Krumhansl, 1993):

> *Physical therapy is an art and science which contributes to the promotion of health and prevention of disease through understanding of body movement. It functions in the prevention, correction, and alleviation of the effects of disease and injury.*

Physical therapy has gained more autonomy than the other allied health professions. A substantial number of PTs operate in private practice, and by 1997, many states provided for direct access for services. For several years running in the mid-1990s, PT was considered to be the most promising, best career position in the United States (among *all* possible jobs), with OT running second at times. In view of the 12–15% shortage in recent years, the field continues to prosper as we approach the new century.

Speech-Language Pathology

The first efforts to alleviate defective speech are traced back to the fifth century BC, when several Greek writers alluded to stuttering, aphasia, and articulation/voice problems. The well-known story of Demosthenes shouting at the sea with a mouth full of pebbles is thought to be the first record of "treatment" for stuttering in the world. An actor named Saryrus was said to be the "speech therapist" who had advised Demosthenes in this approach.

By the mid-1800s, considerable knowledge had been developed about speech in Western Europe (particularly Austria and Germany), and a number of physician-written publications were in existence. The Germanic-speaking areas continued to develop techniques into the twentieth century using a master-mentoring system that restricted the interchange of ideas among the physicians of the practitioner schools.

The American speech movement began around 1910, when several native and naturalized professionals (including Alexander Melville Bell) began reinterpreting some of the theories of their European brethren. The first appearance of speech therapy in schools took place in Chicago and Detroit in 1910, when "speech correction" teachers began serving students; in the next 6 years, Boston, New York, and San Francisco created similar positions. However, it was the Universities of Wisconsin and Iowa that pioneered what would eventually become the field of speech pathology at the higher education level. The first university program was created at the University of Wisconsin in 1915, which granted the first doctor of philosophy degree to Sara M. Stinchfield in 1921. The state of Wisconsin was the leader in the field of speech correction in public schools for many years, particularly at the elementary level. The profession would maintain its association with education for another 30 years.

Because public speaking and speech correction are associated, the beginning of the national association movement for what is now speech and language pathology was challenging. The original conventions were conducted by the National Association of Academic Teachers of Public Speaking, which later became the National Association of Teachers of Speech (NATS) in 1919 and is now known as the Speech Association of America (SAA).

The early challenge for speech correction professionals functioning within the much larger group of peers in NATS was to distinguish the scientific and scholarly study of speech from those interested in rhetoric and public address. Attempts to accomplish this within NATS failed, giving rise to the formation of the American Academy of Speech Correction (AASC) in 1925. AASC was formally sanctioned by NATS 2 years later, and the groups shared conventions for most of the ensuing 25 years. In 1950, AASC assumed its current name, the American Speech and Hearing Association (ASHA). Robert W. West, then the director of the University of Wisconsin speech pathology program (and *second* PhD in the country) is credited with being the active founder of ASHA.

Another icon of the profession was Wendell Johnson, who, among many other accomplishments, succeeded in making the University of Iowa program in speech pathology and audiology the "stuttering capital of the world" (a gross minimization of the total Iowa program, but noteworthy). Johnson, who was himself relatively speechless as a child, served many national and international causes related to speech, hearing, and semantics, and the clinic at the University of Iowa stills bears his name today.

Much like PT and OT, SLP evolved toward acceptance as an ancillary medical service during World War II, when traumatic injuries brought new challenges to the field. Acceptance and reimbursement for services escalated even further in the post-Vietnam era, when legislation funded school programs and geriatric treatment on a broad scale.

In spite of the current specialization and emphasis, these four disciplines have much in common in their developmental histories. The demand for their services came from wars, mental illness, and epidemics. These medical challenges were met by teachers, social workers, and nurses. The result is a fantastic army of multidisciplinary teams performing near miracles on those who would not have walked, talked, eaten, or performed self-care 100 years ago. Hats off to the champions of rehabilitation!

An Alien View

Had you just landed on Earth from Mars and decided to read this book for pleasure, you would most likely say, "ehohni relins boshkatok," which is Martian for "The nurses have it!" Nurses have been organized longer, have the greater numbers, and are better understood by the physicians. As ever-present caretakers, they embody the notion of healing for most Earthlings. Nurses usually know the patients and families better than anyone else and work more with the full spectrum of services on a daily basis. Any sensible Martian would assume that nurses had better pay, hours, and status than their therapeutic counterparts, who, after all, *seem* to have less overall responsibility for the lives of their patients—at least their *in*patients.

You have got it wrong, Mr. Martian. Nurses—even BSNs (Bachelors of Science in Nursing)—start out at salaries lower than COTAs and PTAs, earning less than half of what professional therapists are paid fresh out of school. In the hospitals and nursing homes, they get the rotten shifts and must work their way up through an age-old pecking order to reach day shifts; even then, alternate weekends are usually spent covering shifts. Continuing education money is meager at best (averaging about $75 per year per nurse), and the caseloads approximate criminality.

For 200 years, nurses have been there when the call bell rings, when the cranky physicians make their rounds, and when families come to complain about everything under the sun, including managed care. When a patient passes away, it is the nurse who makes the call deep in the night, long after the therapy team has gone home. Glued to the nursing station in her ever-present white smock, the nurse prays that a dump doesn't arrive late in her or his shift, knowing that it will mean an additional 2 hours to do the admission and accompanying paperwork. Same clothes, same floor, same patients, few new stimuli to break the monotony. Nurses are the continuity factor in medicine. Consistent. Ground zero. Dependable. Tireless.

Consider the therapies. We waltz out of our school programs into cushy *day* jobs, pull down high pay and great benefits, expect the moon for training dollars, and demand modern equipment for treatment. For the most part, our day begins at 8:00 AM and ends at 5:00 PM, save that late admission or drop-in outpatient that keeps us laboring for an extra hour or so. We might have to suffer through an occasional Saturday, or even a Sunday, if we are doing weekend shifts to pay off student loans, but for the most part, we do daytime weekday work. Although we might complain about it, many of us gain variety by working in two or more work sites, getting paid while we drive from one location to another, with mileage reimbursement for a little extra pocket change. We dress in comfortable clothing, go *out* to lunch, and when an educational event pops up, we just reschedule a few things and leave. We have our own office areas (much of the time) and can just close the door when the clamor of the hallway gets too loud. Is it any wonder that nurses feel some resentment?

In Pursuit of the Proper Perspective

Mad at me yet? Angry about these gross stereotypes? Think I'm picking on therapists in favor of nurses? No way. I just want to get your attention. I want to get you inside the heads of those nurses who will never tell you exactly how they feel about the recent invasion of what used to be their sole domain (or is that *soul* domain?). The rationality of these feelings is not the point. You need to understand the perspective of these nurses who are so vital to your work. These are the people who, for decades, did virtually everything for their patients: They bathed them, walked them, fed them, tended to their wounds, and did the nurse's version of ADLs without special title or compensation. Along come these "visitors"—therapists and assistants and RAs and managed care agents and case managers and upper respiratory (UR) staff and respiratory guys and ombudsmen—and the nurses are, metaphorically, pushed to the back of the bus. All of a sudden it seems that everyone else is a specialist, and nurses are relegated to the humdrum generality of daily care. To the nurses, you *in particular* seem overpaid and underworked. You go and come when you please. You get to eat lunch at restaurants. The training time and money you receive is unconscionably high in their minds, and they resent you for it.

On therapy's side of the equation there are counter-resentments. You volunteered or worked for peanuts just to *get in* to your professional school, and the application process was highly competitive, arduous, and expensive. Then you had to work your butt off to graduate. It was the demand for therapists during the golden age that drove up salaries and benefits, not gluttony on the part of the therapeutic disciplines. You can't help it if the sophistication of the science increased reimbursement from Medicare and commercial insurance, it just *did;* therapy works, and that's all there is to it. And it's a good thing! Nurses should be thankful for all the function and independence you bring to their patients. If they followed up your treatment program a little better, recovery would happen even faster. And everyone knows that the professional schools just provide basic training in rehabilitation, not the advanced specialization that comes from healthy continuing education budgets. *Everyone* knows that.

No, not everyone does know that. Nurses also receive basic training in their programs, but they must depend on in-house in-services (or personally funded external workshops) to keep up or advance in the field. Most of them assume that if therapists have a baccalaureate or master's degree, they should know most of what is needed to do the job without all this extra expense. They feel that therapists are unduly pampered, spoiled by the success of their profession, unaware of what it really takes to get a patient well.

I sincerely doubt that a good nurse would ever undermine the health of a patient out of resentment for a therapist. I have never seen it, and I wouldn't expect to. The indignation is a bit more subtle than that. The consequences come in things like delayed calls for orders, cliquish exclusions of therapists from conferences, and unflattering comments to physicians—the kind of bruises that certain nurses can inflict out of unconscious resentment. Not the stuff of all-out war, but just enough to stick in the craw. Therapists can react by withholding needed information or by conveniently leaving a nurse out of a treatment that is normally done in partnership with nursing. The two groups take shots at each other behind closed doors ("those so-and-so therapists, those such-and-such nurses . . ."), but little overt fighting occurs. And so it goes, day after day, a smoldering ember just waiting for enough heat to blow into a major range fire.

Reaching Out for Rationality

There is sufficient irrationality on both sides to keep nursing and therapy at odds, if that is what we want to do. Therapists can walk around like the queens and kings of rehabilitation, knowing that the rehabilitation business has been on a roll, but that isn't going to get the job done. This book is written for therapists, so I must appeal to *you* to reach down deep and try to understand how nurses feel about the loss of control with their patients over the past 2 decades. It is painful for them—particularly the older ones—to feel so ultimately responsible for the patient and yet so limited in what they can actually do. While the doctors may recognize your skill and respect your credentials, most of them still look to nursing for day-to-day continuity with their patients. If you can comprehend the essence of that relationship and bring nursing your wholehearted support and understanding, you will make major strides toward acceptance and a reduction in potential conflict in the future.

Don't accept those sidelong glances and subtle rejections. Get in there and talk to nurses about *nursing*. Find out what makes nurses tick. Eat lunch in the building and create social events that include nursing. Share the history of your discipline, and ask about theirs. Surprise them by letting them know that the first OT was a nurse. Acknowledge their hard work and the contribution it makes to the team. Help a nurse or a CNA with some task that you would ordinarily walk past. Reach out and touch a nurse with respect and kindness. Someone has to make the first move, and it might as well be you!

MORSELS

It has often been said that the sobering reality of working in the Oval Office causes sitting presidents to move to the middle of the political spectrum. There is something about "walking the walk and talking the talk" that moderates the behavior of former candidates who finally carry the big stick after touting their big schtick. I have often wondered if the same thing would happen to nurses and therapists in an exchange program. How would these professionals view each other's work after a week—just a week—of being in the other guy's shoes? Wouldn't *that* be interesting?

16
Conflict Consciousness

A Look at What You'll Learn:

- How to help create a "Yes" work culture
- Why win-win is the best way to approach conflict
- How to assess your emotional capability as an intervener
- The types of conflict that arise most frequently in rehabilitation

You can make a decision right now. You can decide that you don't even like the word "conflict" and just carry on with business as usual. Or, you can read on and say, "Hey, everyone has to deal with conflict in this business. I'm not alone. Maybe I need to think a bit about how I handle the hassles at work. Maybe some of these problems present an opportunity to learn and to show my stuff as a leader. Maybe sometimes I'm part of the problem."

Like time management, conflict resolution has generated its own industry in books, tapes, and workshops. Business rarely operates without interpersonal or intergroup conflicts, and rehabilitation is no different. However, with the possible exceptions of the nurse-therapist dynamic and the ever-present struggle with physicians, there is nothing particularly esoteric about the kind of conflict that arises in our domain. It's the same old struggle about people and power and resources, just as it was when we were 12 in junior high. The only difference now is that we are *supposed* to be grown up.

So, we grown-ups will now take aim at the minefield of conflicts that lay before us as therapist-supervisors. Supervision, performance appraisal, and meetings are the arenas in which most conflict takes place, and you now have a basic platform from which to approach the challenge.

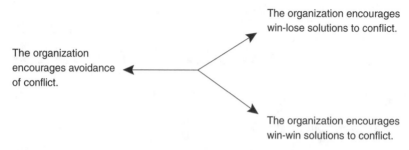

FIGURE 16-1. Organizational approaches to conflict resolution. The policies, procedures, norms, and role-modeling of the leaders in an organization dictate the organizational attitude toward the resolution of conflict. While some companies formalize (as written policy) the corporate philosophy toward the management of such problems, most present a more subtle, day-to-day "way of acting" message, as reflected in their respective history, actions, and reactions.

The "Yes" Culture

Unless you are a single practitioner, you operate in a work culture that affects how conflict is handled. Like most things in business, the tone is set at the top, and the lower layers of the organization follow suit. In fact, when I consult with a new company, I treat the attitude toward conflict as a differential diagnosis, because nothing speaks louder about corporate culture than the way it handles its people problems.

Whether they want to or not, organizations adopt a philosophy toward conflict resolution that is demonstrated by the behavior of its managers. This philosophy can be portrayed in one of three ways, as shown in Figure 16-1.

The avoidance syndrome is probably the worst of the three. The walls can be falling down, yet the norm is to deny that anything is wrong. Old American clichés such as "Don't rock the boat" and "If you can't say something nice, it's better not to say anything at all" come into play. It's business as usual, from top to bottom, and people must simply adjust to whatever is bothering them, or leave. Little or no training is afforded supervisors on conflict resolution, and the confrontation that does occur happens behind closed doors. Boss-types can be heard saying, "Just fix it! I don't want to hear about it!" Serious strife flies right by the supervisors, and meetings are spent darting and dodging around anything that might cause a spat. The focus is on the *business,* as if in some mystical way, the people and their problems are totally divorced from the work. Call it "Numb Are Us, Inc."

The win-lose model is almost as devastating. In this philosophy, conflict is a zero-sum game, and there can be only one winner, be that a person or a team. By definition, the winner can only win at the expense of a loser. Intervention is focused on *who* is right or wrong, rather than *what* is the source of the problem. Supervisors approach conflict with the idea that someone has done something wrong (the loser) in a definite juxtaposition to someone who has done something right (the winner). This philosophy limits the options for everyone involved. Workers at the base of the organization, who are statistically poised to become the losers under this type of system, begin to manipulate around conflicts to assure an occasional victory for themselves. My wife, Barbara, once worked for a company of this type, and I was continually amazed at the stupendous turnover rates that were reported to her. The employees were constantly on edge, just waiting to be accused of having made some kind of awful mistake.

The win-win model is the preferable philosophy in all walks of life. Just as a parent should promote learning, understanding, and growth between sparring siblings, a supervisor should attempt to edify all parties to a conflict, while helping them to resolve the problem. The *problem* should be under attack, not the people, and there should be faith that a fair hearing will always be granted all parties in the dispute. Instead of fixing blame or counterattacking, win-win offers a powerful tool for managing people in the workplace. Farsighted organizations engender such support, because trust in the process creates a comfort throughout, and there is strength in such comfort. The organization is saying to its members, "Yes! We will work through our problems. Yes! You will be heard. Yes! We will learn from our mistakes. Yes! You will continue to be glad that you work here." As a motivator for problem solving, the word "Yes!" is superior to the word "No!"

Emotional Capability of the Supervisor

Now we will narrow the focus on you once again. For our purposes here, I will assume that you want to adopt the win-win approach. You are not blocked from taking on conflict by unrealistic time restraints or company interference. You know that solving human-to-human problems goes with the territory and that avoidance simply makes things worse. You *want* your supervisees to bring problems to you, because interpersonal problems represent unwanted barriers to progress and productivity. You are a leader, and leaders tackle tough problems.

When I think about my personal approach to conflict, the first word that comes to mind is *capability*. Like you, I have bad days, so I must look inward first to evaluate my internal resources before charging out to save the world. I know that I have gone through periods during which I didn't want to help someone else with their hassles. I just didn't feel like it. For whatever reason, I didn't have the energy to deal with another problem—especially if I was involved in that problem—so I avoided. I closed my door. I got busy, suddenly. And of course, like a growing infection, the problem usually got worse while I procrastinated.

Given the luxury of advance thinking, it is a useful exercise to make two preliminary determinations before taking on a conflict. First, are you capable? Are you capable, that day, of getting involved? Can you handle it? Do you have the time, patience, and energy to do a good job? Is this something that should wait until tomorrow?

While total avoidance is undesirable, thoughtful delay can be useful. If you are not prepared to handle a situation and feel that another day will not be fatal, wait! Give yourself the permission to hold off a bit. Usually problems are not as bad as they first appear, and sometimes they can work themselves out overnight. Sometimes they weren't really problems in the first place. It is a judgment call on your part, something that comes with experience.

The second determination is equally as important: Are *you* part of the problem? Did you help cause it? Do you have a role in carrying out the resolution, or are you just an advisor to the process? Are you capable of handling this, or should it be kicked up to someone else because of your involvement? The old Black Panther tenet espoused by Eldridge Cleaver ("You are either part of the solution or part of the problem") may be true about race relations, but it doesn't necessarily fit with supervision. You need not automatically assume that you are part of a problem, nor part of the solution. In fact, that very thought might prevent you from being an effective mediator. There are times when you need to distance yourself from a problem between two other people, including people you directly supervise. It is much harder to find solutions when you project yourself into the problem and complicate the facilitation of the solution.

Causes and Sources

A conflict is a mental struggle or a competitive encounter resulting from opposing actions or views. These actions and views are rooted in our belief systems, our values. Value is the worth, utility, or importance that we assign to ideas, people, or things. As I said in the beginning, I hope that you will hold to your values and bring principle-based management to the workplace. It is a workplace where strong feelings about values are commonplace, because we are dealing with the very lives of our patients, clients, and students. If a physician orders that a deep wound be cleaned with hydrogen peroxide and the PT knows that this can actually *kill* the patient (bubbles in the bloodstream), we have a conflict. When a family member sneaks an orange into a hospital patient that is NPO (*non per os*, not by mouth), we know that the attending SLP has a serious problem to be solved. In both cases, people are acting on their values, but nonetheless, there is a clash because of the actions taken.

The number of potential sources of conflict is endless. However, there is a framework that helps us categorize conflicts for better understanding and strategy. In reviewing the following list, please note that the conflict could occur between individuals, within a group, or between groups. Each category is followed by an example from a real-life rehabilitation situation.

- **Limited resources.** As reimbursement withers, battles over staff time, supplies, and equipment will undoubtedly increase.

Budget struggles between therapy and other disciplines (nursing, teaching, maintenance, etc.) will continue. Management is often asked to intervene. *Example:* As a customer service, your company *always* provided free in-services to the nursing staff on virtually every aspect of therapy; now staffing cuts have reduced that to a minimum. The DON wants to know why.

* **Control.** Your professional independence is eroding. Increasingly, you are a visitor on someone else's turf. You request orders of nurses who interpret them to doctors; neither person totally understands the therapy, and yet they make decisions that affect your work. Who controls the patient? As your company becomes more decentralized and middle management shrinks, who runs the show at the facility level? The practice act and clinical pathway say that treatment should be done this way, but the department head says that productivity requirements dictate otherwise: To whom or what do you listen? The HMO's case manager automatically limits every patient to six or fewer visits from a single discipline, and you have a complicated stroke patient who will need at least 8 weeks of PT, OT, or SLP to show improvement. *Example:* A patient with frail skin desperately needs a wheelchair seat cushion. The local managed Medicare HMO refuses to pay for both the cushion and the visit needed to install it properly, even though it would be covered under traditional Medicare benefits. When you press the issue, they say, "Get Medicare to state in writing that they cover this supply, and we'll allow it." Fat chance of that ever happening!

* **Misunderstandings.** Miscommunication, failure to listen, inadequate documentation, and late information can all lead to misunderstandings. Fortunately, this is one of the easier categories to fix if it isn't a chronic problem. *Example:* An SLP tells the transportation staff that she needs a patient taken over for a barium swallow test today. At 2:00, she storms in, angry that the patient is still in his room. By *today,* she meant *this morning,* because the tests always occur before noon. The van driver didn't understand that.

- **Trust and confidence.** In a multidisciplinary environment, we must be able to depend on each other. A breech of faith or failure to follow through can leave lasting uncertainty that leads to further conflict. *Example:* A young PT recommends home exercises for a wheelchair-bound 10-year-old paraplegic who is fairly noncompliant. The exercises are painful, and the parents complain to the teacher who says, "Oh don't pay any attention to her, she's just a kid."

- **Personality conflicts.** We all have our personal styles. Some of us talk too much, some not at all. Some of us see the glass as half empty, while others see it as half full. Working so closely together, we get on each other's nerves. In our own selfish way, we expect other people to be like us. They aren't. We even assign nasty personality traits to *groups*: that *stupid* dysphagia team, that *dumb* third floor staff, those *boneheads* over at company X. If they aren't part of us, there must be something wrong with them, right? And we're grown-ups? *Example:* A senior staff OT continually blasts a competing therapy company for their poor clinical practices. "Those guys are a bunch of crooks," she cries. "I'm surprised that they can get anyone to work there!" Two months later, she becomes their new site manager and loves them.

- **Inadequate performance.** We touched on this one several times in the sections dealing with supervision/coaching and performance appraisal. When expectations are mismatched, not clear, or simply not met, we get conflict in the vertical sense. Depending on your station in the company, this could be the inadequacy of an individual or of an entire organization. *Example:* A PT sees some 15–18 patients a day in his outpatient clinic. The aide is supposed to have new charts ready to go to speed the documentation process. For some reason, every second or third chart is missing a form. The excuses are many and varied, but the incomplete work continues for weeks on end.

- **Work structure.** This is a biggie. With all the changes that are occurring, redesigning has altered the landscape considerably. New teams form almost weekly, and job assignments shift like the wind. Those who had aides to support them are suddenly out looking for a friendly CNA to help with a transfer. Caseloads have increased, reporting assignments have changed, and now they want to redo all the forms. School therapists who used to have a small cadre of buildings to cover now have an entire district to oversee. So much change! Too much change! *Example:* The veteran PT who debrided in the burn unit for *years* is now holding the gait belt for geriatric patients in the nursing home. She has asked for a transfer back to the hospital at every supervisory meeting for the past 6 months, to no avail. She is *not* a happy camper.

- **Failure to cooperate.** Oooh! None of us likes this one! Whether it is a therapy team that refuses to meet productivity goals or a nurse-therapist duo that decides not to get along after mediation, it feels like betrayal. Ongoing noncooperation cannot be excused by misunderstandings or change or a lack of alignment if people set their minds to digging in and acting out. Cooperation and collaboration are at a premium right now, and overt noncompliance evokes strong reactions from managers. *Example:* A regional manager is charged with equalizing the caseloads across outpatient, home-care, group home, and nursing home services to balance the hours for the therapists and assistants, who are paid hourly. The staff is cross-trained in all areas, so clinical skills and documentation capability are not a problem. Census drops in every sector, except the group homes. Instead of calling the regional manager to share the caseload, the group home staff runs up 18.5 hours of overtime in a single week, while the remaining staff averages 32.75 regular hours per therapist for the same week. Result: extra expense to the company and inadequate paychecks for the therapists who were sent home. Conflict!

• **Feelings.** Much as we might try, we carry our feelings around like butterflies in a bag, hoping that they won't fly out and get stepped on. It's hard to avoid emotional involvement in this kind of work, especially when frustration and exhaustion combine to erode our defenses. Hurt, anger, fear, and guilt lurk just below the surface as we make our way through the maze of decisions and compromises each day, testing our values against those of the outside world. *Example:* A PTA on her second affiliation presents an in-service to the PT team. The subject is the use of pneumatic pulsation devices to reduce edema for the promotion of wound healing. She is very excited about her presentation, having spent nearly 15 hours in preparation. Three therapists show up, and two of them spend the entire lunch hour catching up on late documentation. The third misses 20 minutes of the talk to take a personal phone call. The PTA cuts the presentation short and leaves in tears. She spends the next 3 years badmouthing the company that employed her discourteous "mentors."

• **Sense of status.** Although we might like to think otherwise, we are all conscious of status. People look at your dress, your title, and your car, and then judge you accordingly. When I walk through a hospital wing or a nursing home wearing a suit and a name tag, I am often stopped by patients wanting to know if I am a doctor. "No," I usually answer, "But I play one on TV!" This little vignette might not be the best example of status, but it makes the point. Overblown status and rigid pecking orders— the hyperbole of inflated egos—are not particularly attractive, but we know they exist, because we see them every day. On the other hand, legitimate status orientation—like supervisory structure—serves a good purpose in an organization, because it defines lines of authority and accountability. *Example:* An OT transfers to the rehabilitation unit from bedside ortho med and is surprised to find out that the COTA there is the strongest clinician on the unit—so strong, in fact, that she is consulted on all evaluations of neurologic patients, even by the PTs! The OT complains to her program manager. "A COTA shouldn't have that much influence," she whines.

Isn't it amazing how these scenes play themselves out in so many settings so many times? In the next chapter, we look at the way employees deal with conflict, while learning some valuable intervention strategies.

MORSELS

For me, the biggest conflict that occurs when I am intervening with battling employees is not what is going on between them, but what is going on within me. Each time I sit down with them, I must consider a number of important decisions:

- Should I contribute to the discussion or just observe for a while?

- How do I avoid taking sides?

- How can I find "neutral" words to avoid fueling the fire or sounding biased?

- Do I really have a bias for the solution?

- What are the long-range implications of this intervention? Am I establishing myself as a useful mediator or setting up a dependency by getting involved?

- Does the content have merit, or is this just a power struggle?

- How can I avoid getting my own feelings and solutions mixed in with *their* problem?

- How do these two people stack up in their respective attitudes and behaviors in this session? Who is being the most reasonable? the most rational? the most cooperative? the most resistant?

- Can we resolve this in one session?

- Will I have to make a decision *for* them?

- If this is true incompatibility, with no resolution, will I have to separate these two? Who will leave?

- How can I bring this to some conclusion?

This type of mind-talk should be going on in your head every time you sit down to help resolve a conflict. If it isn't, you are going to drive the session toward *your* solution, which might not be the *best* solution—not to mention the bad precedents you create for the future. If you have *no* internal conflict in such situations, you probably already know the result you want going in. That might be fine, in some scenarios. However, I would personally worry if *my* answers were always required to solve the interpersonal problems beneath me. Personal empowerment for my employees comes when they struggle a while and then discover and implement solutions that work for them.

17
Intervention

A Look at What You'll Learn:

- How most people respond to conflictual situations
- How to diffuse tense situations using the management principles
- Why active listening is such a powerful tool
- Specific language techniques for addressing conflicts
- New ways to look at old conflicts

Time for the home stretch. Knowing that a problem is bound to be right around the corner, you take a walk around the block and contemplate what you have learned. A little self-analysis has refreshed your sense of personal values at work, and you know that long-term solutions are preferable to short-term fixes. You know how to hire, supervise, coach, evaluate, and meet with groups of staff in ways that promote professional growth, personal maturity, and profitable productivity. Only conflict management stands between you and supervisory immortality.

If you have been exposed to the various personality inventories (Minnesota Multiphasic Personality Inventory, Myers-Briggs, Jungian Types, Fundamental Interpersonal Relations Orientation B, Psycho-Geometrics, etc.), you know that there are some clever ways to categorize social styles. Although I am not particularly enamored of some of the labels, they do serve a good purpose in fostering an understanding of people and how they are likely to react in conflict or crisis. Such tools are also helpful in hiring and assembling teams, because they remind us of the value of diversity.

Response to Conflict: Fight, Flight, or Insight?

As you continue your stroll, a thought emerges: *If everyone—including us—responded to conflict in an even-tempered, rational fashion, collaboration and compromise would prevail, and management would be a snap! I wouldn't have to read this section of the book!* Unfortunately, resolution doesn't always happen that way. Let's take a look at the negative reactions that do tend to show up.

I will once again wax physiologic. When a mammal is threatened, the sympathetic nervous system is activated, and the fight-or-flight mechanisms take over. The endocrines kick in, blood floods to the muscles and brain, body temperature rises, and the pupils dilate: The body is prepared to take action through rapid movement, either forward or backward. When an employee encounters a conflict, similar but subtler responses are observed as the attempt to survive emerges. In addition to the neuromuscular responses, we see associated behaviors that also represent fight or flight. Bob Phillips, in his book *The Delicate Art of Dancing with Porcupines,* has classified these fight-or-flight behaviors into a grid called "The Four Responses to Conflict." As shown in Figure 17-1, an adaptation of Phillips's concept, fightlike responses are further divided into people who withdraw or give in, while flight reactions include those who dominate or attack.

I am certain that you have seen these reactions in yourself and others in both your public and private lives. When you went through the four response types, who were you thinking of, yourself or other people? How *do* you react to conflict most of the time? Are you pensive? quiet? expressive? active? a fighter? a flyer? How about the people you work with—your core and extended team members, the doctors, the patients, the family members? Are you chasing them around trying to work things out with them, or are they in your face?

The setting in which conflict occurs makes little difference, because the social style of people is fairly consistent, be it in a one-to-one struggle or within a group or family. Other classification systems use such terms as *dominators* and *aggressives* for the fighters and *avoiders* and *peacemakers* for the flyers, but the basic ideas are similar.

Flight Reactions	Fight Reactions
▼	▼
WITHDRAW	DOMINATE
Tend to become less assertive; more controlled; hold in their feelings; keep quiet; don't share ideas; avoid; dodge; escape; retreat from other people and undesirable situations.	Overly assertive; autocratic; unbending; over-controlling; demanding; strong-willed; imposing thoughts and feelings on others.
GIVE IN	ATTACK
Give in to others; keep the peace; reduce conflict; agree when secretly disagreeing; strong desire to save the relationship, even when personally hurt.	Attack others emotionally; attack ideas; use condemnations and put-downs to discredit; strong emotions.

FIGURE 17-1. Four responses to conflict. Behavioral reactions to conflict attend the physiologic responses that prepare human beings for fight or flight during conflict. By reading and recognizing such responses, sensitized supervisors can reduce their own reactions to these predictable symptoms in order to proceed more efficiently with effective interventions. (Adapted from B Phillips. The Delicate Art of Dancing with Porcupines. Ventura, CA: Regal Books, 1989.)

When you shake it all down, the basis of fight-or-flight responses is *fear*. It may come out as anger, argument, anguish, or abandonment, but the bottom line for all us fighting animals under the sun is fear. We are afraid that we don't know enough. We might make a mistake. We could be embarrassed. We could become dominated by someone stronger. We're even afraid that *we* might dominate and then feel guilty for doing so! If you grasp this concept and believe it—for yourself and those you work with—you will begin to understand how to manage conflict. People simply don't open up and get creative when they are scared. They attack, dominate, withdraw, or give in. Therefore, we must alleviate as much fear as possible.

Management by intimidation, with rare exception, does not work. As a leader, your job is to reduce the threat, redirect the focus toward problem solving, and then help facilitate the solution.

You round the final corner and head back to work, wondering who will hit you with the first conflict. By now, you know that problems aren't special: They're normal.

Strategic Diffusion

Conflict can bring out the best or the worst in a supervisor. Let's reflect on the management values that were covered in Chapter 2 to help you be your best:

- Honoring the Golden Rule
- Keeping one's integrity intact
- Valuing teams and teamwork
- Being congruent in your work and personal life
- Edifying
- Assuring consistency
- Being useful and valued
- Sharing love

Walking into a bonfire that was kindled by fear is much easier with such principles under your belt. You have the self-assurance that people just want to be treated fairly, honestly, and lovingly and that you will be consistent and helpful in helping them to work out their differences.

The most powerful tool in the de-escalation of a conflict is listening. *Active* listening. This technique is basic training for psychiatrists, psychologists, social workers, and group facilitators because they regularly deal with the charged emotions of personal and interpersonal conflict. I have used it in several examples thus far without giving it a specific label. The crux of active listening is acknowledg-

Table 17-1. Active Listening Prompts

I see.
I understand.
I don't understand.
I see what you mean.
Tell me more about . . .
So you feel that . . .
Can you clarify for me . . .
Let me summarize what I think I heard . . .
So it was your understanding that . . .

ment—acknowledgment that a person has truly been heard. It sounds simple, but it takes thought and practice.

Thomas Gordon, the father of Parent, Teacher, and Leader Effectiveness Training, taught thousands of people (myself among them) about the difference between the *content* and *feeling* of what people say when they speak in an emotional way. Most of us are conditioned to hear and then acknowledge content, as if we had the balance adjustment on our stereo turned to one side. By learning to decode the message and offer a response that acknowledges both content *and* feeling, we take a huge step toward helping a person to become more rational. This is particularly true with children, because emotion so often overpowers fact. And, because professionals tussling over an issue so often act like children, active listening is a pertinent skill for intervention.

Active listening *in the midst of conflict* involves a series of non-threatening, nonjudgmental questions; attempts to clarify; verifications of content; summaries of the problem; and validations of feelings in an effort to keep someone talking. Table 17-1 offers some useful phrases to help with actively listening to someone with a problem.

Note that I have stressed *conflicts* and *problems* as the context for using active listening in the previous paragraphs. Because the technique is such an effective method of communication, it can begin to spill over into normal human discourse and become problematic. When people don't have a problem to reveal (or if they do, but it's none of your business), they don't want to feel interviewed by a friend or a colleague. Active listening is basically an interviewing technique, but one that should be reserved for *problem-based* situations. When it becomes a habit in normal conversation, it sounds like contrived sincerity, and you begin to sound phony. Working in the mental health field in the late 1970s, I saw a lot of this during breaks, lunch, and social events and found it very annoying. Learn it, use it, practice it, and revere it for its wonderful value. Then leave it where it belongs—in the middle of conflictual situations.

To take a look at effectiveness technique and some active listening that helps drive it, I will pull an example from an encounter I had once with a PT. This woman was upset with me for writing a first-warning letter for her personnel file after a serious problem had arisen in a nursing home. I had worked with her for several years, and her reputation for outbursts had been addressed by previous supervisors in private conversations and in performance appraisals. The most recent blowup with a DON could have cost the company a therapy contract. For our purposes, I will name the PT Jenny Smith, or JS. Please understand that exact reconstruction of the conversation is impossible, but this is the gist of it:

JS: *I feel that your letter was wrong and unfair, and I'm upset.*

GM: *You look upset, Jenny, and I'm sorry that I had to write it. Was it the letter itself that upset you?*

JS: *No, not really. I guess the stuff in it was accurate enough.*

GM: *So you don't understand my purpose in writing it?*

JS: *Not really. I just don't see what the big deal was. We [Jenny and the DON] got in an argument about that new nurse, and I couldn't help myself. I got pissed. When I feel strongly about something, I have to let people know. I thought it was over and done with, you know, forgotten.*

GM: So you were surprised when it came up again, a month later?

JS: Yeah! And I thought this woman was my friend! I've worked with her for years. We go all the way back to the hospital together.

GM: Sounds like you feel a little betrayed.

JS: That's putting it mildly. She knows me. She knows I mouth off once in awhile. But she also knows darn well that that new guy is totally lost. He doesn't know what he's doing! All I did was say the obvious!

GM: I know, and from what other people have said, your observation was probably correct. But how do you think the DON felt, having you criticize her new hire right in the middle of a meeting like that, where nurses and therapists could hear everything?

JS: Embarrassed, I guess. And threatened. But that doesn't change who he is! He's a disaster! He's dangerous! Every nurse in that building would tell you that!

GM: I know, and I respect the fact that you are so good about trying to protect your patients. But do you understand why I felt I had to write the letter? Do you see that when you sounded off like that at the DON, it put the contract at risk, and that I was afraid of losing that contract? You have to be more diplomatic with key people.

JS: Oh, I don't know. I suppose so. I know I should keep my big mouth shut sometimes. But it's hard when you know you're right.

GM: I know it is. But we've been over this same thing several times. It was about the only problem area cited in your last appraisal, and it nearly cost us the contract. I had to let you know the seriousness of the situation. You are an exceptionally good clinician, but these verbal assaults cause you relationship *problems. Without those relationships, you can't help the patients. And if we lose the contract, none of us can help the patients. You can't play if you're not in the game.*

JS: *I know, you're right. I'm still not happy about it, but I'm glad we talked.*

Notice the dynamics that begin this conversation. As is typical of these situations, Jenny began with fairly short, blocky sentences, indicative of how bottled up she was. This is typical of conflictual encounters. The first thing I do (I always do) is make strong, unwavering eye contact. It is very important for this person to know that I am truly *engaging* him or her in conversation. I am not off somewhere, thinking about other staff or patients or DONs or budgets, with my attention divided. My eyes say that I am listening, hearing, and wanting to understand.

As I asked questions and acknowledged Jenny's feelings and content, she spoke more. This represented the venting portion of our talk. Sometimes that is all that a person wants or needs, and you perform a service by actively promoting such catharsis.

As our discussion moved along, I attempted to shift Jenny's anger away from the letter (and the male nurse) toward what she had said to the DON that caused the problem that resulted in the letter. I let her talk around that subject for awhile to diffuse the emotions before hitting the nail on the head.

This meeting continued for about 15 minutes. During the portion that you just read, there were eight exchanges: Jenny spoke eight times, and I spoke seven times. If you divide the exchanges down the middle and analyze each half of the conversation, you will notice a considerable difference in the number of words spoken by each of us in the two halves of the conversation. In the first half, Jenny spoke a total of 92 words, while I spoke 49 words, a ratio of about 2 to 1. The reverse ratio was true in the second half, wherein my count was 188 words, and hers was 107. By listening actively, I encouraged Jenny to express *her* feelings before I voiced any thoughts of my own. Until she did that, she was in no position to accept my observations, thoughts, or suggestions for future behavior on her part.

Too many times, supervisors try to open a meeting like this with force and anger, and the person leaves the meeting never having learned from the experience. If you can use active listening to ground an upset employee long enough to get out their initial beef, you will have plenty of time to express your own thoughts and feelings later.

Because this incident was the most recent of many, the letter was a necessary formality but of no less importance than this meeting. Jenny left feeling that she had been heard and treated fairly, even if she disagreed about the presence of the letter in her personnel file. I also felt better, because I knew that Jenny understood that her verbal transgression was the focus and that I had made no overall indictment of her abilities as a therapist.

One of the things I like about the Gordon Effectiveness Training approach to communication is that it has a describable structure. You first learn to really listen to what you are hearing, then to decode it carefully, and finally to structure your responses in a specific manner.

For an example of decoding, let's look at a few of Jenny's remarks. The first statement was "I feel that your letter was wrong and unfair and I'm upset." Notice that I looked past the accusation that I was "wrong and unfair" and focused first on her being upset and then on the letter itself. By affirming Jenny's emotion (instead of my own, which I could have projected as anger), I eventually found out that she felt most strongly about being betrayed by the DON. This led to discovering how angry Jenny was toward the new nurse and, finally, how fearful she was about the fate of her patients, who stood to be served by this man. This emotional baggage—betrayal, anger, and fear—is what Jenny brought into our meeting in the form of anger.

Now let's look at the structure of *my* responses in this conversation. My first few sentences were short clarifying questions or statements confirming that I was listening while I gathered further information: "Was it the letter itself that upset you?" "So you don't understand my purpose in writing it?" "So you were surprised when it came up again, a month later?" "Sounds like you feel a little betrayed." These are invitations to speak more, to release more emotion. The word "you" is in every sentence, not "people like us" or "she" or "they." This is purposeful in active listening, because you are trying to get at the real feelings of the person in front of you. In the last statement, I avoided saying, "Sounds like *she* betrayed you" to keep the focus where I wanted it—on Jenny.

Strategic Feedback

We turned the corner in this discussion when Jenny admitted that she understood how the DON might have felt ("Embarrassed, I guess. And threatened."). At that point, I began the educational process of explaining the consequences of Jenny's mistake in behavioral terms. This approach to structuring one's sentences is a basic strategy in conflict resolution, where you must be sure to identify (1) the behavior that you want to change, (2) the negative consequences of that behavior on you or others, (3) how you feel (felt) about that behavior, and (4) what you want done for remediation. The key sentence in the conversation with Jenny was "Do you see that (1) **when you sounded off like that** at the DON (2) **it puts the contract at risk**, (3) **and that I was afraid of losing that contract?** (4) **You have to be more diplomatic with key people.**"

1. The behavior I wanted to change = *when you sounded off like that*

2. The negative consequences of the behavior = *it puts the contract at risk*

3. How I felt about the behavior = *and that I was afraid of losing that contract*

4. What I wanted done for remediation = *You have to be more diplomatic with key people.*

About now you might be saying, "This is too complicated! I can't think about all that at once!" Actually, you can, but it takes practice. If

Table 17-2. Structuring Strategic Feedback

Step 1: Listening	Capture content and feeling
Step 2: Responding	Offer questions, prompts, clarifications, and summaries of the problem(s)
Step 3: Behaviorally based statement	Communicate both that the unwanted behavior will equal a consequence and what your feeling about that consequence is
Step 4: Remediation instruction	Communicate what you want done to prevent similar consequences in the future

you have kids or a roommate, give it a try the first time they come in with a problem. Sequence your interaction with the steps shown in Table 17-2, and stand back, because you will most likely get an earful.

This type of "strategic feedback" is most pertinent when you are part of the conflict, as I was with Jenny. However, as shown in Figure 17-2, you encounter a variety of conflict scenarios in your daily life as a therapist-supervisor, and the supervisor-employee is only one example. When you are *mediating* between individuals or groups (such as the employee-employee or team-team scenarios shown in Figure 17-2), use steps 1 and 2, and then work toward extracting steps 3 and 4 from the warring parties. These last two steps are accomplished by going back and forth, asking about how people feel and what they want done. It never fails to amaze me how people begin to problem solve more maturely once they diffuse the emotional component of the conflict equation. It's like watching a fast forward of *The Wonder Years.*

Other Conflict Concepts

If you apply the management principles, listen and speak selectively and effectively, and use the facilitation skills from Part IV for group and intergroup conflicts, you will have 98% of your interventions covered. The remaining 2% of the game (at least from my perspective) is covered by the following tips:

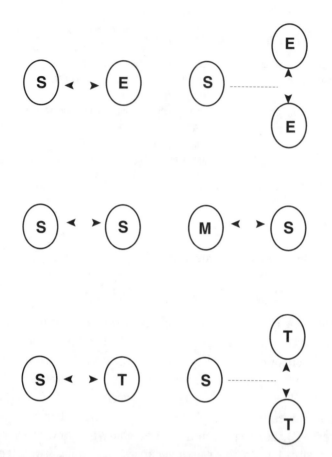

FIGURE 17-2. Conflict scenarios. The therapist-supervisor faces conflicts with individuals, between individuals, between teams, with peers, and with persons of superior status in the organization. While different strategies must be applied to the various combinations, the most common starting point in all conflicts is effective listening on the part of all parties to the conflict. (S = supervisor; E = employee; T = team; M = manager/administrator.)

- *Avoid unnecessary interventions.* Establish a firm policy with your team about *your* intervention in *their* squabbles. Explain, in a nice way, that you want them to always attempt to work out their interpersonal/intrateam problems on their own. Go over the strategies that they should follow when they can't work things out, including going over your head (with your knowledge) if necessary. Actually, I like to see all organizations publish such a policy on conflict resolution, because it is healthy and helpful.

- *Discourage triangulation.* This is an offshoot of the first tip. Triangulation occurs when you come to tell me about a problem you have with someone else, inviting me to become part of the solution. This happens to all employees, supervisory or not. Redirection to the proper source—the person with whom the problem exists—is the ticket. Be particularly aware of this phenomenon when an employee from another team approaches you for help instead of going to his or her own supervisor. Resist the temptation to intervene; you might as well swallow drain cleaner as get involved in someone else's problem.

- *Don't overdo it.* Stick to the core people when working through a conflict. Don't invite the world to your intervention party thinking that there is strength in numbers—there is *complication* in numbers if too many people (or the wrong people) are included. Large groups stifle process, and confidentiality faces a greater test.

- *Establish ground rules when mediating.* This is a repeat reminder about aligning expectations in what could be a tense situation. This is not normally required in a one-to-one intervention, but it could become necessary. We once had a woman at CMT who was notorious for jumping up and running out of the room every time she became upset; she would represent the exception to the rule.

- *Begin with the end in mind.* If you can, carve out some time to think about where you want to go with an intervention before starting up. Sometimes the venting of anger or learning is all that you can expect in certain conflicts because of time or situational limitations. Don't try to move a mountain before you've even reached the foothills. Also, don't be discouraged by a lack of resolution; sometimes things just don't work out, no matter what you do.

- *In selected situations,* overstate *the animosity.* This is a technique I learned in working with my children. In certain situations, when I suspect that the conflict is really just a spat rather than a battle, I will exaggerate the situation in an effort to get people to stand back for a moment to look at their own silliness. With the kids, I say something like, "Boy, you guys really *hate* each other, don't you? I can't believe how much you *hate* each other right now!" In tiny voices, they always say, "Well, it's not really hate. I'm just mad, that's all." Adults are just bigger kids, and they respond the same way.

- *Make sure you understand the problem before seeking solutions.* Nothing is more embarrassing than taking a swan dive into the wrong issue. Let people talk. Let them fight a bit, if necessary. Summarize the gist of the conflict, and have the person/group validate your summary before proceeding.

- *Summarize the learning that has taken place.* This is particularly true if the result of the intervention didn't feel much like resolution. Summarization has more impact if you avoid the parental twist ("Do you understand what you have learned here?") in favor of estimating your own personal growth ("I know I've learned something through all this.").

- *There are times when* you *must decide.* In spite of your best efforts, there are times when intervention and due process just don't cut it, and you must make a decision that resolves the conflict. Also, when a true crisis exists, requiring immediate action, you can't be spending time processing people's feelings. That time may well come, but not until the immediate emergency is dealt with.

- *Praise the survivors.* Showing the courage and perseverance to stick it out through a crisis deserves reward. Be sure to affirm people's participation after you've been through a struggle together. Something like, "I appreciate you guys trying to work out your differences like this; it feels good," is all it takes to remind employees of their hard work while encouraging them toward resolutions in the future.

Talking about conflict resolution as if it were a single, definable skill would be like calling curry a spice. Curry is a collection of spices, emanating from a consistent base of four spices (coriander, turmeric, cayenne, and cumin) to as many as a dozen. If your conflict resolution recipe includes four basic tools (ethical management values, group facilitation technique, active listening, and strategic feedback), you will definitely give your employees something to chew on.

MORSELS

In their book, *Swim with the Dolphins,* Glaser and Smalley point out that children laugh an average of 400 times a day, whereas adults manage a meager 15. As a supervisor, you can help your people lighten up the workplace in so many ways by choosing to see the humor rather than the gloom in conflict. Humor has a way of downsizing problems and hastening creative solutions. I just can't stress that enough!

18
Post-Master (In the AfterTASC)

I sincerely hope that the philosophy and techniques shared in this book prove useful to you as a therapist-supervisor. Even more, I hope you will listen to your heart and go forward in directions that inspire you to achieve your greatest potential. If clinical work is your true love, stay there and enjoy the rewards that treatment brings you. If you find supervision particularly challenging and rewarding, there is always room for new blood in middle management should you want to move in that direction. If you like treatment and management equally, rehabilitation is one of the few industries in which you can probably find a leadership position that satisfies both needs. Whatever you do, take your management principles along and live by them religiously.

Several times, in the body of this book, I suggested that you pause to take a personal inventory before proceeding with something new. Here, in the afterTASC, I suggest it once more. This time, however, the inventory is for you to take after you have had a little experience. After having served as a therapist-supervisor for awhile, ask yourself the following questions:

- How do I feel about the responsibility of a leadership role?

- Do I look forward to organizing and facilitating my team meetings, or are they a tiresome responsibility?

- Does this dual role (therapist and supervisor) leave me exhausted all the time? If so, which role is the most tiring?

- Do I find that I am chronically behind, unable to keep up?

- Do I enjoy managerial problem solving?

- Do I look forward to encounters with those who bring me problems?

- Do I feel energized after performance appraisal sessions?
- Do I enjoy being the messenger and interpreter for upper management?
- Is it unduly stressful for me to say "no" to my employees? Do I constantly fret over such decisions?
- Am I good at getting productivity from the staff I supervise?

Your personal answers to these questions can be helpful in making career decisions. If they imply that supervision is not your strong card, then don't pursue a position in middle management, where the pressure to account for the work of others only gets worse. Stay where you are. Apply the principles. Adjust to the new era by improving the management of yourself above all else. Be a happy TASCmaster!

In closing, I want to leave you with a brief review of the salient points of this book. These things were said many ways, in many places, because a useful book, like a useful person, should be integrated and consistent.

- Therapists are severely pressed for time, and although not necessarily inclined to do so, they should attempt to develop skills in supervision and coaching. The new era will bring increased pressure to be effective as a leader at the line-staff level, and those who are prepared will be more competitive in what will become a saturated market. While the management role requires a new focus, much of it uses skills that therapists already possess, such as assessment, monitoring, and the measurement of outcomes.

- Effective management is principle-based, and the most basic of the principles is the Golden Rule.

- The therapist-supervisor is a key attendant of the boundary between management and labor, a role with inherent conflicts. Supervisors who bring an honest, open, humble, and responsive approach to this role will engender trust on both sides of the power differential; this trust then becomes the foundation for building strong teams and successful individuals.

- Much of management—from hiring to retiring—is an ongoing process of aligning the expectations of the employee with those of the organization and its appointed leaders. When this alignment process is attended by a philosophy that allows decision making at the lowest possible level, employees assume more responsibility and ownership and are thereby empowered. Vertical and horizontal empowerment strengthens the fiber of any organization.

- Rehabilitation is a relationship-based business, and the ability to engage, develop, and maintain key relationships is critical to effective self-management and efficiency. In every aspect of management (hiring, supervising, coaching, facilitating meetings, ending employment, and managing conflict), those who can listen well and strive to truly appreciate the perspective of others will, in the end, be better positioned to succeed as leaders.

- The demands of the modern workplace threaten to strip us of our humanity by forcing us to *become* our work. Against this tide, we should stand firm in all facets of our lives, with a resounding commitment to regain that which we have nearly lost in the rush to succeed: balance. Employees who come to work with a sense of balance are employees who go home with a sense of accomplishment.

Suggested Reading

Abbott M, Franciscus M-L, Weeks ZR. Opportunities in Occupational Therapy Careers. Chicago: NTC Publishing Group, 1988.

Baron RA. Behavior in Organizations. Boston: Allyn & Bacon, 1983.

Block P. The Empowered Manager. San Francisco: Jossey-Bass, 1987.

Committee to Study the Role of Allied Health Personnel. Allied Health Services: Avoiding Crises. Washington, DC: National Academy Press, 1989.

Costa P, Widiger T. Personality Disorders and the Five-Factor Model of Personality. Washington, DC: American Psychology Association, 1994.

Covey SR. The Seven Habits of Highly Effective People. New York: Simon & Schuster, 1990.

Creasia JL, Parker B. Conceptual Foundations of Professional Nursing Practice (2nd ed). St. Louis: Mosby, 1996.

Donahue MP. Nursing: The First Art. St. Louis: Mosby, 1985.

Douglas ME, Goodwin PH. Successful Time Management for Hospital Administrators. New York: AMACOM, 1980.

Ellis JR, Hartley CL. Nursing in Today's World. Philadelphia: Lippincott, 1995.

Glaser C, Smalley BS. Swim with the Dolphins. New York: Warner Books, 1995.

Gordon T. Leader Effectiveness Training. New York: G.P. Putnam's Sons, 1983.

Hopkins HL, Smith HD. Willard and Spackman's Occupational Therapy (5th ed). Philadelphia: Lippincott, 1978.

Institute of Financial Education. Supervisory Personnel Management. Chicago: Institute of Financial Education, 1988.

Kraegel J, Kachoyeanos M. Just a Nurse. New York: E.P. Dutton, 1989.

Krumhansl BR. Opportunities in Physical Therapy Careers. Chicago: NTC Publishing Group, 1993.

Larkins PG. Opportunities in Speech-Language Pathology Careers. Chicago: NTC Publishing Group, 1988.

Lynch D, Kordis PL. Strategy of the Dolphin. New York: Fawcett Columbine, 1990.

Martin D. TeamThink. New York: E.P. Dutton, 1993.

Miller D. Living, Laughing and Loving Life. Mukilteo, WA: Winepress Publishing, 1997.

Paul S, Paul C. Tough/Nice. Evergreen, CO: Delta Group Press, 1988.

Phillips B. The Delicate Art of Dancing with Porcupines. Ventura, CA: Regal Books, 1989.

Szilagyi AD, Wallace MJ. Organizational Behavior and Performance (3rd ed). Glenview, IL: Scott, Foresman & Company, 1983.

Tavris C. Anger: The Misunderstood Emotion. New York: Simon & Schuster, 1982.

Tubbs SL. A Systems Approach to Small Group Interaction (5th ed). New York: McGraw-Hill, 1995.

Williamson DL. Group Power. Englewood Cliffs, NJ: Prentice-Hall, 1982.

Wolff L, et al. Fundamentals of Nursing (7th ed). Philadelphia: Lippincott, 1983.

Appendices

Appendix 1
Me and Supervision

Instructions: To discover some of your thoughts and feelings about supervision, complete the following sentences.

Compared with patient care, supervising others seems _____
_____
_____
_____

The thing that worries me the most about supervision is _____
_____

In supervising, I am (would be) most comfortable when _____
_____

My biggest weakness as a supervisor is (would be) _____
_____

I (would) want my supervisees to describe me as being _____
_____

I (would) want my supervisors to describe me as being _____
_____

In leading a meeting, it is always hard for me to _____
_____

One aspect of supervision that I really don't like is _____
_____

As a supervisor, I would describe my style as . . . (**circle all that apply**)

quiet strength	thoughtful	verbal	withholding
confident	hesitant	erratic	demanding
critical	open	scattered	nurturing
organized	inspirational	confrontive	predictable
misunderstood	forceful	dependable	persuasive

Appendix 2
Key Incident Journal

Name: _____ Appraisal period: _____

Date	Description of Incident	Discussed with Employee (✓)

Appendix 3
Structure of a Good Performance Appraisal Instrument in the Rehabilitation Industry

I. Basic data. To be a useful document for the personnel file, the performance appraisal form should include the following basic data:
   Employee name
   Supervisor(s) name
   Title of position*
   Period of appraisal (3 months? 1 year?)
   Date of hire

II. Performance categories. To obtain a thorough appraisal of performance for the period, at least five areas should be evaluated:
   Teamwork
   Professionalism
   Work quality
   Productivity
   Evaluation and treatment

III. Performance criteria. Within each category, criteria should be created to achieve the proper measurement of performance. The language of these performance criteria reflects the values of the company and goals it wishes to achieve. The following are some examples for each of the categories listed above:
   A. Teamwork
      1. Communication
      2. Flexibility
      3. Contribution to the team(s)
      4. Management of conflict

---

*If more than one position has been occupied by the employee during the period, the most recent position title should be entered.

     5. Demonstration of respect for others

B. Professionalism

     1. Personal integrity

     2. Commitment

     3. Punctuality

     4. Tact

     5. Personal appearance

     6. Pride in the work area

     7. Professional growth (pursuit of education)

C. Quality

     1. Compliance with policies and procedures

     2. Timeliness

     3. Follow-through

     4. Innovation

     5. Documentation

     6. Customer service

     7. Outcome orientation

D. Productivity

     1. Efficiency

     2. Prioritization

     3. Enthusiasm/energy

     4. Ability to work under stress

E. Clinical criteria

     1. Treatment-related

        a. Resourcefulness

        b. Observation skills

        c. Appropriateness of choices

        d. Communication with relevant parties

        e. Reimbursement knowledge

     2. Safety and compliance

        a. Sufficiency of knowledge

        b. Compliance with rules

     3. Assessment/reassessment

        a. Pertinence of collected information

        b. Thoroughness

        c. Integration of information

    4. Reimbursement/documentation
      a. Qualifying patients
      b. Describing treatment plans and progress
      c. Differentiating treatment types
    5. Supervision
IV. Rating scale. Most rating scales contain five to seven levels of performance. The following is a six-level system, beginning with the lowest level:
    Unacceptable—When performance is clearly and consistently below stated expectations and little or no effort has been made to improve performance
    Deficient—When performance does not meet expectations, but the potential for improvement has been demonstrated by attitude and effort
    Fair or improving—When performance is acceptable at times but inconsistently so. Performance is in need of development in order to reach the acceptable level of competency
    Good—When performance consistently meets or occasionally exceeds expectations; provides service at a level that would be expected of a professional who is qualified and experienced
    Very good—When performance frequently exceeds expectations; service provision is given above and beyond what would normally be expected
    Exceptional—When performance is consistently above expectations; extra efforts and initiative are unique and sustained over the review period
V. Scoring and financial reward
    A. Scoring. If increases in pay or bonuses are to be tied to performance appraisal scores, an objective, defensible merit system should be installed. Such a system should vary from company to company, depending on the corporate values, the focus of the work, and the finances. Some companies choose to set up a standard scoring system for which the merit increase percentages are set each year, according to the financial health of the company at the time. The following is an example of a scoring-merit system for a medium-sized rehabilitation company:

Performance	Level Equivalent Score
Unacceptable	0
Deficient	0
Fair or improving	3
Good	4
Very good	5
Exceptional	6

1. Supervisor scores. If these numbers are applied to the criteria from the five performance categories listed earlier, four merit increase range levels can be created from the total score. Because there were 36 criteria in the example, the highest possible score is 216 (36 × 6). The threshold for each level is totally arbitrary, according to the preferences of the company. The following model for classifying the supervisor's total appraisal score uses the percentile approach that is familiar to most of us from school testing; it is offered merely for the purpose of demonstration and not necessarily for actual use.

Level	Point Range	% of Total Possible
I	194–216	90–100%
II	173–193	80–89%
III	151–172	70–79%
IV	130–150	60–69%

Thus, an employee scoring a total of 183 would fall into level II in this model.

If this score from the supervisor's ratings is the *total* score (i.e., no other sources are to be added), the merit increase is applied in the amount equivalent to level II (see B. Merit pay increase equivalents, on the facing page).

2. Self- and peer scores. If self- and peer evaluation scores are to be included, all scores (including those from the supervisor) must be weighed before being summed to the *total* score. The following example weighs scores from three

sources of performance appraisal: the supervisor (weighted at 70%), the self (weighted at 15%), and the peer (also weighted at 15%). Note that the original totals in this case, before weighing, are 185 (supervisor total), 174 (self-appraisal total), and 188 (peer appraisal total).

Source	Original Total	% Weight	Final Subtotal
Supervisor	185	70	130
Self	174	15	26
Peer	188	15	28

Total score: 184

This score, the weighted total of three sources of input, would place the employee at level II (173–193) in the model shown above.

B. Merit pay increase equivalents. The final step in a merit-based pay increase system is to apply the score level to an equivalent merit pay increase amount. As shown above, the score can be calculated from a single source of performance appraisal (usually the supervisor) or from multiple sources (supervisor + self + peer + other). Once again, the actual percentage of the increase equivalents is determined by the company, not by industry standards (which do not exist) or the examples shown here (which might have been typical in the early 1990s).

Level	Merit Pay Increase %
I	7–10%
II	5–8%
III	4–6%
IV	0–4%

An employee with a score of 184 would fall into level II under this scheme, with a potential pay increase within the range of 5–8% of the annual salary in effect at the time of the performance appraisal. A *range* of percentage increases is preferable to a single number, because it allows the supervisor to account for certain variables in giving the merit increase. For example, if self-evaluation is included in the total score, and it is quite low compared with the peer and supervisor scores (as is often the case), the supervisor might choose to give the employee a 7% increase for a level II score of 184 rather than a 6% increase. On the other hand, if the self-scoring was far above the peer and supervisor scores, the supervisor might choose to give a 5% increase as opposed to a 6% increase. A number of additional variables affect this decision, not the least of which is attitude of the employee being evaluated. If an employee has demonstrated an eagerness to learn new skills and improve on deficiencies, the flexibility of the merit pay *range* affords the supervisor the opportunity to acknowledge such efforts. Conversely, there is the employee who turns to gold the final 3 weeks of the appraisal period after 49 weeks of mediocre performance; choices within the equivalent range also accommodates the supervisor's need to remind employees that a year lasts a full 52 weeks.

VI.   Performance action plans. This is the goal-setting section of the performance appraisal instrument, wherein the supervisor and supervisee discuss growth, remediation, and the future. Many companies simply use a blank page for this important activity to maximize creativity. The following is a format (complete with examples) that can be used:

Issues	*Action Plan*
1. Incomplete documentation samples	Training from supervisor; random chart to be reviewed each month
2. Complaints from nursing staff about attitude	Complete assigned reading; attend conflict resolution course; attempt to establish better relationships within extended team
3. Treatment of stroke patients	Attend NDT course; complete assigned reading; join stroke team

VII. Sign-off sheet. The final page should include space for comments from both the supervisor and the employee, as well as signature and date lines. A preprinted statement—such as the one that follows—is often included on the signature page to qualify the signature:

Your signature does not necessarily indicate agreement with the appraisal, only that it has been discussed with you. You are obligated to acknowledge the appraisal if your supervisor has discussed it with you.

The act of securing the signature is particularly important, because performance appraisals often become part of the legal paper trail, and a signed, dated form indicates that the discussion occurred. Also, the employee should always receive a complete copy of the signed document.

Appendix 4
Time Will Tell: A Self-Survey

Instructions: Circle the response that best describes you, and total the numbers at the bottom.

	3	2	1
A. Promptness			
I am rarely late for anything at work.	3		
I am occasionally late.		2	
I run late much of the time.			1
B. Preparedness			
I feel prepared for my work most of the time.	3		
Sometimes I find myself ill-prepared for my work.		2	
I am often ill-prepared for work.			1
C. Personal pace			
The pace of my work day is even and comfortable.	3		
I feel pressured by time restraints but not rushed.		2	
I feel that I am constantly rushing at work.			1
D. Crises			
It is rare that I deal with a crisis at work.	3		
I deal with an occasional crisis at work.		2	
I respond to crises at work on a regular basis.			1
E. Planning			
I budget time to plan each week.	3		
I plan sporadically, not regularly.		2	
I rarely take the time to plan.			1
F. Scheduling			
Rarely, if ever, do I fail to meet my appointments.	3		
Missed appointments occur occasionally.		2	
Foul-ups on appointments occur for me quite regularly.			1

3 2 1

G. Filing
   I rarely have difficulty finding my paperwork.   3
   There are times when I cannot find my paperwork.   2
   Lost or misplaced paperwork is a regular issue for me.   1

H. Delegation
   I give work to other people on a regular basis.   3
   I give some work to others, but could give more.   2
   I have difficulty giving work and do most things myself.   1

I. Handling hard copy
   I rarely touch mail or paperwork more than once.   3
   I shuffle paper around a bit, but it's not a great   2
      problem.
   My mail and paperwork are a mess, and it's a   1
      real problem

J. Completing documentation
   I am rarely more than 3 days behind on   3
      documentation.
   I run between 3 and 7 days behind in my   2
      documentation.
   I am almost always more than a week behind in   1
      my documentation.

Total score ____

Appendix 5
TASC Terms: The Language of Management and Supervision

Note: Tr = traditional; GM = Morse-coined.

Administrative

Administration (Tr): Activities emanating from or having to do with the highest levels of the organization; usually associated with presidents, vice-presidents, CEOs, COOs, CFOs, CAOs, executive directors, directors, administrators, superintendents, or principals who have significant authority.

CAO (Tr): Chief administrative officer. Sometimes used interchangeably with CEO or executive director; handles overall executive functions, including contract management.

CEO (Tr): Chief executive officer. Has overall executive power to run the organization. Hired by owners or board of directors. Sometimes called executive director or administrator.

CFO (Tr): Chief financial officer. Has fiscal responsibilities for organization, including finance and accounting.

Mission statement (Tr): The written purpose of an entity, usually an organization. Can be a single sentence, a paragraph, or a lengthy tome describing the purpose, philosophy, and product or service of the entity. Personal and departmental mission statements are also seen occasionally.

Pro forma (Tr): Latin for "as a matter of form." A focused budget created to study the viability of a project or a purchase. Contains revenue, expense, and profit figures over time.

Return on investment (ROI) (Tr): A financial analysis of the revenue (or other measures, such as market share) to be gained or lost on an expenditure. Normally used for capital investments such as real estate and equipment, but can be applied to an investment of time or personnel to a project. Evaluation of ROI is a good way to look at the effectiveness of meetings.

Strategic planning (Tr): An orchestrated effort at establishing goals, objectives, action plans, and assignments for short-term or long-term achievements. Generally an administrative activity created for the overall organization, but can be departmental in focus.

Conflict Resolution

Active listening (Tr): A set of verbal and nonverbal techniques used to encourage a person or group to share thoughts or feelings. Uses prompts, questions, and encouragement to bring forth what would normally be withheld. Recommended when the other person is experiencing conflict.

Strategic feedback (GM): The act of providing verbal feedback regarding behaviors or acts that you want changed in a strategic fashion. A blocked statement identifies the aberrant behavior, its negative consequences, and how you feel about those consequences. It should be followed by an indication of the remediation you expect.

Win-win (Tr): A conflict resolution philosophy oriented toward maximizing gains by both parties to the conflict. Requires an effort for the mediator to remain neutral in the intervention.

General

Empowerment (Tr): A work situation in which the employee takes responsibility and feels a sense of ownership for the work, the job, and the organization. A philosophy of management that allows for such dynamics among workers.

Expectancy-valence theory (Tr): A work theory (developed by Victor H. Vroom) that assumes that people are motivated to work when they have the expectancy that the work environment will provide them with valued outcomes that they seek.

Expectation alignment (GM): A set of management strategies designed to assure the alignment of expectations between the employee and the job, the supervisor, and the organization. If adopted by a company, it is applied at every opportunity, including hiring, supervision, meetings, and performance appraisal.

Extrinsic motivation (Tr): Worker motivation based on external outcomes that are gained as a result of work performed. Salary and benefits are examples of extrinsic motivation.

Ground rules (Tr): Established methods of procedure and behavior for a group, meeting, or conflict resolution session. Generally brought by the leader (or mediator) and shared at the beginning of a session.

Interdependence (Tr): Within a team or group, reliance on fellow members to be responsive and to pursue commonly held goals and objectives. The ability to depend on a fellow team or group member.

Intrinsic motivation (Tr): Worker motivation based on internal outcomes gained from work performed. Solving problems and feeling satisfied for having served others are examples of intrinsic motivation.

Leader (Tr): One who sees the global picture and assumes responsibility for generating plans and action.

Multidisciplinary (Tr): A team or a service composed of workers from several areas of professional emphasis (therapists, nurses, social workers, etc.). Sometimes called *transdisciplinary.*

Peer (Tr): Traditionally described as an equal of the same rank and of similar ability, value, or quality. In this book, *peer* is used to describe a fellow team member or other worker whose support and input are valued, regardless of his or her discipline or status.

Productivity (Tr): The yield of work from time spent working, usually expressed as a percentage. In rehab, the norm ranges from 65% to 75%, depending on the setting and other variables. Known as the

"*P*-word," it has become the focus of much consternation on the part of therapists in the late nineties.

Requisition (Tr): A form requesting approval for a purchase, a rental, or a new position.

Time study (Tr): A detailed record of time spent on work tasks by a single employee or a team over a designated period of time, such as a day, a week, or a month. Normally in increments no less than 15 minutes.

Human Resources

ADA (Tr): Americans with Disabilities Act. Federal legislation created in 1990 to protect disabled persons from discrimination. Requires employers to make certain accommodations (physical and procedural) for disabled employees.

COBRA (Tr): The acronym for Consolidated Omnibus Budget Reconciliation Act of 1985. Federal law that provides for a potential 18-month extension of medical and dental benefits for employees separated from employment if they choose to pay premiums.

Corrective action (Tr): Actions taken by an employer to remedy performance deficits on the part of an employee. Can include counseling, retraining, reassignment, suspension, demotion, and warning letters to the personnel file.

Decreasing duration (GM): A term coined for an applicant whose resume reflects a pattern of decreases in the duration of successive work positions.

EEO (Tr): Equal Employment Opportunity. Federal civil rights law that provides equal opportunity for employment to American workers. Overseen by the EEOC (the Equal Employment Opportunity Commission).

FTE (Tr): Full-time equivalent. Commonly used by managers to describe the hours allocated to a full-time work position. Normally a 40-hour-per-week job, which equates to 2,080 hours per year (52 weeks × 40 hours). A half-time position would be described as a 0.50 FTE.

Human Resources Department (Tr): Interchangeable with *Personnel Department*. Provides support services related to employment, such as recruitment, screening, interviewing, hiring, benefit management, corrective action, promotion/demotion, and separation.

Job description (Tr): Written detail of the design of a work position; usually includes qualifications, responsibilities, duties, and physical/mental requirements.

Job enlargement (Tr): A job redesign technique intended to increase the number of activities within the job duties.

Job enrichment (Tr): A job redesign technique intended to increase the responsibilities and ownership in the outcome of a job.

Job jumpers (GM): A term coined to describe a person whose resume reflects a pattern of jumping from one work position to another without significant tenure with any one employer.

Motivational appraisal (GM): An inflated performance evaluation given to a less-than-satisfactory employee in the hope that good scores will increase motivation; not a recommended practice.

Orientation (Tr): The process of familiarizing a new employee with all aspects of the job. It should include the job description; introductions to key people; assignment of benefits; and education about the job, team, assigned facility, supervisory arrangement, and company.

Paper trail (Tr): Formal written record of important activities, usually in sequential form. In the human resources context, the paper trail constitutes any source of written information on an employee that could be used in a court of law for personnel-related actions. The most common sources are the personnel record and the supervisor's personal file on the employee.

Performance appraisal (Tr): Formal review of work performance for an employee. Normally accomplished in face-to-face meeting between supervisor and employee with a copy of written record placed in the personnel file. Can be conducted at any time, but traditional period is after 3 months in a new position or annually. Also known as performance review, annual review, or work assessment.

Probation (Tr): Antiquated term for initial work period (usually 3 months), in which employee performance and attitude are evaluated to determine if continued employment is recommended. Due to legal and motivational complications, most companies now use the term *evaluation period* in lieu of *probation*. *Probationary period* is also used to describe the work period immediately following corrective action.

Reduction in force (Tr): Politically correct term for layoffs (usually more than one person). In personnel jargon, the action is called *RIFFing*.

Reverse performance appraisal (GM): Any system that formally provides regular feedback from supervisee to supervisor on the quality of supervision, the job, and the organization.

Review period (Tr): The period of work time in which performance is being appraised in an evaluation (e.g., 3 months, 1 year).

Separation from employment (Tr): The act of discontinuance from the employer-employee relationship (e.g., resignation, termination, retirement).

Suspension (Tr): The temporary removal of an employee from the active performance of job duties. Normally invoked for violation of company rules and regulations (e.g., life-threatening act, positive drug screen) or during an investigation of an employee's behavior.

Termination (Tr): Forced separation from employment of an employee. Also called *termination for cause*.

Turnover (Tr): The act of losing employees from employment through termination or resignation. The *turnover rate* is the number of employees lost per year compared with the number of positions available, usually expressed as a percentage. A high turnover rate is often indicative of internal problems in the company.

Meeting Management

Agenda (Tr): Verbal or written list of topics to be covered in a meeting. Can be distributed in advance or at the time of the meeting. If given in advance, should include date, time, and location.

Facilitator (Tr): The person in a group or meeting charged with enhancing the flow of discussion. Can also be called *leader*.

Group dynamics (Tr): The interplay of members of a group or meeting. Also used to describe the study of such interplay.

Group process (Tr): The manner in which a group works within itself, particularly in solving problems.

Housekeeping (Tr): Helpful information dispensed by the leader or facilitator of a group when it first convenes in a new location (location of bathrooms, food, phones, etc.).

Management theater (GM): A phenomenon in which every activity performed by a manager is keenly observed by supervisees.

Minutes (Tr): Official written record of a meeting or conference; can become a legal document in many circumstances.

Redirection (Tr): A group facilitation technique that either changes the subject or the emphasis of the discussion on a subject.

Teamwork-bound terminology (GM): Language that promotes teamwork and ownership in a process or project being developed by a team; includes terms such as "we," "us," and "ours."

Think-sync (GM): The tendency for a homogeneous group to have similar thoughts, ideas, or solutions to problems.

Organizational Structure

Boundary management (Tr): The management of the interface between subsystems within a larger system, such as an organization. Supervisors and middle managers perform such functions, because they work the borders among teams and between line staff and upper management.

Core team (GM): The team with which the employee identifies most or which the supervisor designates as the primary team for a given employee.

Extended team (GM): The multidisciplinary team that goes beyond the therapists. In a hospital or nursing home, this would include nurses, social workers, physicians, activities/TR, case managers, and other regular members of the group.

Matrix supervision (Tr): A structure that provides for more than one supervisor for a single employee. Normally occurs when the employee is providing services to more than one setting or is involved in a special project or program that requires special supervision. In these cases, the primary supervisor should take charge of the performance appraisal and receive input from the other supervisors in the matrix.

Middle management (Tr): Levels of management between administration and line staff with formal management titles. In rehabilitation, such positions as regional manager, program manager, program coordinator, or rehab services manager apply.

Organizational chart (Tr): A graphic representation of organizational structure. Useful in demonstrating lines of accountability and authority, as well as the relationship of teams.

Senior staff (Tr): A title (often with compensation) for a therapist whose expertise, tenure, and leadership in the discipline warrants recognition and additional responsibilities as a mentor.

Span of control (Tr): The number of employees under the direct supervision of a single supervisor, manager, or administrator.

Span of jurisdiction (GM): The number of employees for which a supervisor or manager is responsible. A middle manager could have a span of control over four therapists, each or whom supervises two additional people; this would make for a span of jurisdiction of 12 for the middle manager.

Stakeholders (Tr): Persons having a financial or emotional investment in the success of a company.

Stockholders (Tr): Persons who own shares in a company.

Supervision

80/20 Principle (Tr): A ratio used for several purposes in management. One informal theory is that a group performs best when it is composed of 80% compliant members and 20% noncompliant. Another says that 80% of the work is accomplished by 20% of the workers. Both are sometimes called Pareto's Principle or Pareto's Law.

Approachability (Tr): An overall quality of openness in a supervisor that invites discourse from others. A pleasant demeanor and obvious desire to be helpful foster approachability.

Coach (Tr): One who provides regular step-by-step instruction and feedback to enhance the performance of a private individual, worker, or athlete. Sometimes associated with mentoring, should be future oriented.

Dream-making (Tr): A term for those individuals who support others in the pursuit of their dreams. Coined by motivational speaker Dan Miller.

Edification (Tr): To instruct and help build the mind of another person, especially morally or spiritually. Goes beyond mere education by seeking and finding the special qualities in an individual and reinforcing them through support and positive feedback.

Hyper-helper (GM): An employee whose excessive need to help is detrimental to her- or himself, the team, or the patient.

Mentor (Tr): One who takes a special interest in tutoring another in a designated area of study. In rehabilitation, this is normally a clinical application. Also associated with coaching and senior staff.

Parent trapping (GM): A phenomenon wherein a boundary manager fails to take ownership or responsibility for a decision or message from a higher level in the organization. This approach to laying blame elsewhere serves to paint higher-ups in a negative light, thereby "trapping" them in a parental role.

Passive-aggressive personality disorder (Tr): A pervasive pattern of passive resistance to demands for adequate social and occupational performance, beginning by early adulthood and present in a variety of contexts. Used less formally in this book to describe employees who refuse direct confrontation, deny responsibility for their actions, and attempt to solve interpersonal problems by going to a third party.

STUPORvisor (GM): A supervisor who ignores her or his assigned employees in favor of performing clinical work; usually responds only when problems occur.

Supervisee (Tr): One whose work is overseen by another person of higher status in the organization. In this book, *supervisee* is used when discussing assistants and techs.

Supervisor (Tr): One who oversees the work of another person. In this book, *supervisor* is normally used in conjunction with the *supervisor-therapist*: physical therapists, occupational therapists, and speech-language pathologists.

SUPERvisor (GM): A supervisor who tries to be the end-all and be-all of answers and solutions for his or her employees. By smothering others with this support and knowledge, he or she extinguishes the joy of discovery.

Time Management

Delegation (Tr): The act of assigning tasks or responsibilities to another person, usually a subordinate.

Pyramid of proficiency (GM): A systematic approach to attacking a hierarchy of external variables that consume time and thereby reduce efficiency. The pyramid contains three triangular faces, called the *three faces of ease*.

Quadrant II* (Tr): One of the four quadrants of the time management matrix from Stephen Covey, used to describe activities that are

---

*From The Seven Habits of Highly Effective People. Copyright 1989 Stephen R. Covey. Reprinted with permission. All rights reserved.

important but not urgent. A good self-manager attempts to choose quadrant II activities, which include prevention and relationship-building efforts. In this book, the pursuit of quadrant II activities is considered to be essential to effective time management.

The three faces of ease (GM): The three triangular faces of the pyramid of proficiency, a system used to attack external variables that consume time. A hierarchical system of organizing the variables from the most difficult (at the point of the triangle) to the easiest (at the base).

Urgency addiction (Tr): The tendency to treat most activities as urgent; a crisis-oriented work mentality.

Index

Arrogance, 113–114

Balance, importance of, 30–31
Budget Reconciliation Act of 1997, 4

Calendars and organizers, 144–145
Cheyenne Mountain Therapies (CMT) survey of therapists, 6–9, 11
Coaching. *See* Supervision and coaching
Confidentiality, 105–106
Conflict, 241–251
    approaches to resolution of, 242–243
        avoidance syndrome, 242
        win-lose model, 242–243
        win-win model, 242–243
    causes and sources of, 245–250
        control, 246
        failure to cooperate, 248
        feelings, 249
        inadequate performance, 247
        lack of trust and confidence, 247
        limited resources, 245–246
        misunderstandings, 246
        personalities, 247
        sense of status, 249–250
        work structure, 248
    and emotional capability of supervisor, 244–245
    responses to, 253–267
        active listening, 256–262
        fight or flight, 253–256
        strategic feedback, 262–263
        use of ethical management values for, 256
    scenarios for, 263, 264
    terminology, 292
    tips for managing, 263–267
Consistency, as management principle, 24–26

Continuing education, 24
Corrective action, 73, 78, 129–131. *See also*
        Termination, employee
Covey, Stephen R., 147–151
Customers
    primary vs. secondary, 39–43
    of therapist-supervisor, 41–42

Delegating, 101–103, 104–105
Documents, drafting of, 203–204

Edification, as management principle, 23–24
Elimination of position, 132
Empowerment, 34–39. *See also* Relationship management
    and organizational design, 38–39
    and problem solving, 34–38
Encounter groups, 178–179
Expectancy-valence theory, 65
Expectation alignment, 65–74
    company expectations, 67, 68
    employee expectations, 70
    in exit interviews, 73–74
    in hiring, 72
    in orientation, 72
    in performance appraisals, 73
    in promotion and demotion, 73
    realignment, 69–70
    in supervision and meetings, 72–73
    within corrective action, 73

"Family," organizational structure as, 50–54, 61–62
Family of origin, and dysfunctional behavior at work, 54–58
Firing. *See* Termination, employee
Foundation skills, 1
Friendships in workplace, 48–50

Golden Rule, as management principle, 17–18
Gordon Effectiveness Training, 256–262

Group dynamics, 177–183. *See also* Meetings
 inevitability of process, 186–187
 influence of "group movement" on, 178–179
 power of, 180–181
 process vs. content, 182–183
Group Power, 180–181
Growth as a manager, 59–62

Hiring, 75–92. *See also* Interviewing; Orientation for new employees
 corrective action, 78
 interviews and reviewing resumes, 77
 job orientation, 78
 job requisition, 76
 performance appraisal, 78
 recruitment, 76
 seeking resumes or applications, 76–77
 selecting finalists, 77
 separation, 79
Human resources terminology, 294–296
"Hyper-helpers," 55, 56

Ignorance, 113–114
Integration, as management principle, 21–23
Integrity, as management principle, 18–19
Interviewing, 79–87. *See also* Hiring; Orientation for new employees
 group, 85–87
 pre-interview tips, 79–81
 tangential questions for, 83–85

Job descriptions, 158

Key incident journal, 123, 279

Leadership, reflecting on, 13–15
Love, as management principle, 28–30

Management principles, 16–30
 being useful and valued, 26–28
 consistency, 24–26

Management principles—*continued*
  edification, 23–24
  Golden Rule, 17–18
  integration, 21–23
  integrity, 18–19
  love, 28–30
  teamwork, 19–21
Management training, 8–9
Meetings, 168, 171–210
  agenda for, 190–193
  avoiding total failure in, 175
  boredom and, 174
  choosing members of, 189–190
  closure for, 208
  dysfunctional people and, 205–208
    documenters, 207–208
    dominators, 205–206
    latecomers, 205
    procrastinators, 206–207
    "snipers," 206
    underminers, 207
  ground rules for, 195–196
  group, types of, 183–184
  group dynamics and, 177–183. *See also* Group dynamics
  location of and food for, 195–196
  outcomes of, 184–186
    changes in the organization, 186
    confidence in the meeting, 186
    coordination, 185
    improved interpersonal relations, 185
    planning, 185
    solutions to problems, 184–185
  setting tone of, 195–199
  terminology, 297
  ways to direct, 199–201

anger, 201
  clever moves for dying meetings, 200–201
  humor, 200
  prompting quiet participants, 200
  redirection of discussion, 199–200
written supports for, 201–205
  charts, 202–203
  draft documents, 203–204
  memos, 204–205
  minutes, 201–202
  supplementary reading, 202
Mentoring, 97
Minutes, of meetings, 201–202
"Molting process," 59–62
Motivation, extrinsic vs. intrinsic, 66

Nurses, 221–239
  advanced practice, specialties of, 226
  animosity of toward therapists, 237–238
  disadvantages of jobs for, 235–236
  formal degrees of, 225
  professional heritage of, 222–227

Occupational therapists
  formal degrees of, 229
  professional heritage of, 227–230
Omnibus Budget Reconciliation Act of 1984, 3
Organizational structure, 43–48. *See also* Relationship management
  as a "family," 50–54, 61–62
  span of control, 44, 46
  span of jurisdiction, 44, 47
  terminology, 297–299
Orientation for new employees, 87–91. *See also* Hiring
  introduction to company, 90
  introduction to facility, 89
  introduction to job, 90–91

Orientation for new employees—*continued*
   introduction to supervisor, 91
   introduction to team, 89
   personal and professional expectations, 88

Paper trails, 126–127
   and corrective action, 131
Paperwork, managing, 169–170
"Parent trapping," 58–59
Passive aggressive behavior, 56–58
Peer performance appraisal, 121–122
Performance appraisal, 115–128
   delivery of, 125–126
   goal setting during, 118
   job enlargement and enrichment, 118–119
   motivational, 126–127
   paper trails and, 126–127. *See also* Paper trails
   as realignment opportunity, 117–119
   resources for, 119–124
      hard-copy, 123–124
      peer appraisal, 121–122
      performance appraisal instrument, 120, 281–287
      self-appraisal, 121
   reverse, 127–128
   writing style for, 124–125
Physical therapists
   formal degrees of, 232
   professional heritage of, 230–233
Pyramid of proficiency, 154–170. *See also* Time management
   ease of access, 158–164
      and approvals, 159–160
      to information and documentation, 163–164
      and patients and clients, 160–161
      to treatment resources, 161–163
   ease of communication, 164–168
      and extended team, 165–167
      and nonurgent, nonimportant activities, 165

and team meetings, 168. *See also* Meetings
and technology, 167–168
ease of influence, 155–158
  over company/department variables, 156–157
  over facility variables, 155–156
  over job design and priorities, 157–158

Reduction in force, 132
Relationship management, 33–62. *See also* Empowerment
  with customers, 39–43
  family of origin and, 54–58
    "hyper-helpers," 55, 56
    passive-aggressives, 56–58
  friendships, 48–50
  growth as a manager, 59–62
  and organizational structure, 43–48. *See also*
    Organizational structure
  "parent trapping," 58–59
Resignation, 132, 133–135
Retirement, 133
Reverse performance appraisal, 127–128

The Seven Habits of Highly Effective People, 147–151
Speech-language pathologists, professional heritage of, 233–235
Splinter skills, 1
Stage fright, 31–32
Supervision and coaching, 93–114
  acts of good management, 109–113
    aiming at the middle, 111–112
    celebrating victories, 109–110
    complimenting work, 109
    cultivating creativity, 112–113
    dream-making, 110–111
  balance of, 98–99
  "cowboy" approach, 101
  definitions of, 96–98
  delegating, 101–103

Supervision and coaching—*continued*
   flexibility in, 99–100
   and mentoring, 97
   responsiveness, 94–96
   SUPERvisors vs. STUPORvisors, 94–95
   terminology, 399–300
   worst transgressions in, 103–108
      delegating inappropriate tasks, 104–105
      failure to follow through, 103–104
      failure to respect others, 107–108
      indecisiveness, 106–107
      violating confidentiality, 105–106
Suspension, 132–133

T-groups, 178–179
Teamwork in rehabilitation, 213–220
   conflict and, 219–220
   as management principle, 19–21
   problem of belonging to multiple teams, 215–219
   team identity, 214–215
   variety of people in, 213–214
Termination, employee, 129–136
   corrective action, 129–131. *See also* Corrective action
   resignation instead of, 133–135
   session for, 135
   terminology, 131–132
Termination for cause, 132
Time management, 137–170. *See also* Pyramid of proficiency
   evolution to self-management, 142–146
      early mechanical stage, 142–144
      late mechanical stage, 144
      outcome-based stage, 146
      planning-based stage, 145–146
      schedule stage, 144–145
   self-survey for, 289–290
   terminology, 300–301

"urgency addiction," 151
urgency vs. importance, 147–151
To-do lists, 144
Training, management, 8–9
Treatment resources, lack of access to, 161–163
Turnover rates, 136

"Urgency addiction," 151

Values, personal vs. professional, 15–16
Vocational divorce. *See* Termination, employee

Williamson, David L., 180–181